A Collection of Stories from Black Families

On the Front Porch

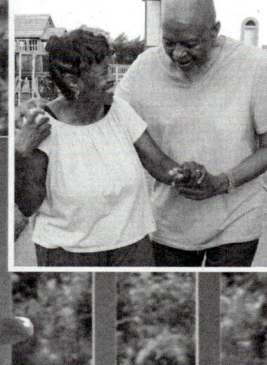

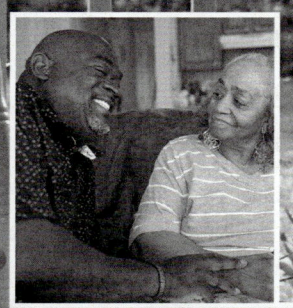

Caring for a Loved One Living with Dementia

DR. PAULA S. DUREN

A Collection of Stories from Black Families

On the Front Porch

Caring for Loved One Living with Dementia

ISBN: 9780988283466

Photos: New City Photographic, Michael Sarnacki

Copyright © 2023

All rights reserved. No part of this book may be reproduced or utilized in any form or by any means, electronic or mechanical, including photocopying, recording or by any information storage and retrieval system, without permission in writing from the Publisher. Inquiries should be addressed to 24342 Ridgeview Dr, Farmington Hills, MI 48336.

First Edition

A Collection of Stories from Black Families

On the Front Porch

Caring for a Loved One Living with Dementia

Acknowledgments

It is with great pride that I reflect on those that have been so gracious to me as I am engaged in this labor of love – Caring for Caregivers.

Life changed directions when both of my parents were diagnosed with dementia-related diseases. I made a commitment that their last days would be the best days of their lives. I am thankful for the love shared, lessons lived and the gifts given to me by my parents. I honor them first for allowing me the privilege of walking with them on life's last journey. We laughed, cried and fussed but never gave up on each other. Their beauty blossomed in my heart with every step of the journey.

Thank you to the wonderful families that trusted me to come into their homes and openly shared their caregiving experiences. I view our time together as a special gift. In return, we have tried to create a product that respects and honors you and your families.

There are so many on the team that contributed to the production of this book and brought their special gifts to the table while respecting those we touched.

Thank you Diane Palmer for being my lifelong friend, who brought this book to life. You believed in our vision of caring for caregivers from day one.

Michael Sarnacki thank you for beautifully capturing the moving imagery of each family we have displayed in this book.

Ellen Columbia thank you for listening deeply to the stories to support the writing.

Special thanks to the editorial, administrative and graphic design team members at DP Marketing Strategies, Inc.

Thanks to my wonderful Universal Dementia Board of Directors for always offering encouragement and guidance.

David Costa, as a board member and lifelong friend I thank you for donating the first financial gift that made my "proof of concept" possible. You believed in me and confirmed the proof already existed.

Special thanks to you Peter Lichtenberg for being the first to confirm our program, "Caregivers Passage through Dementia" would add great value to the field. You and your team were a tremendous help in establishing our program as evidence based.

Special thanks to the Ralph Wilson Foundation/Community Foundation of Southeast Michigan for supporting this project.

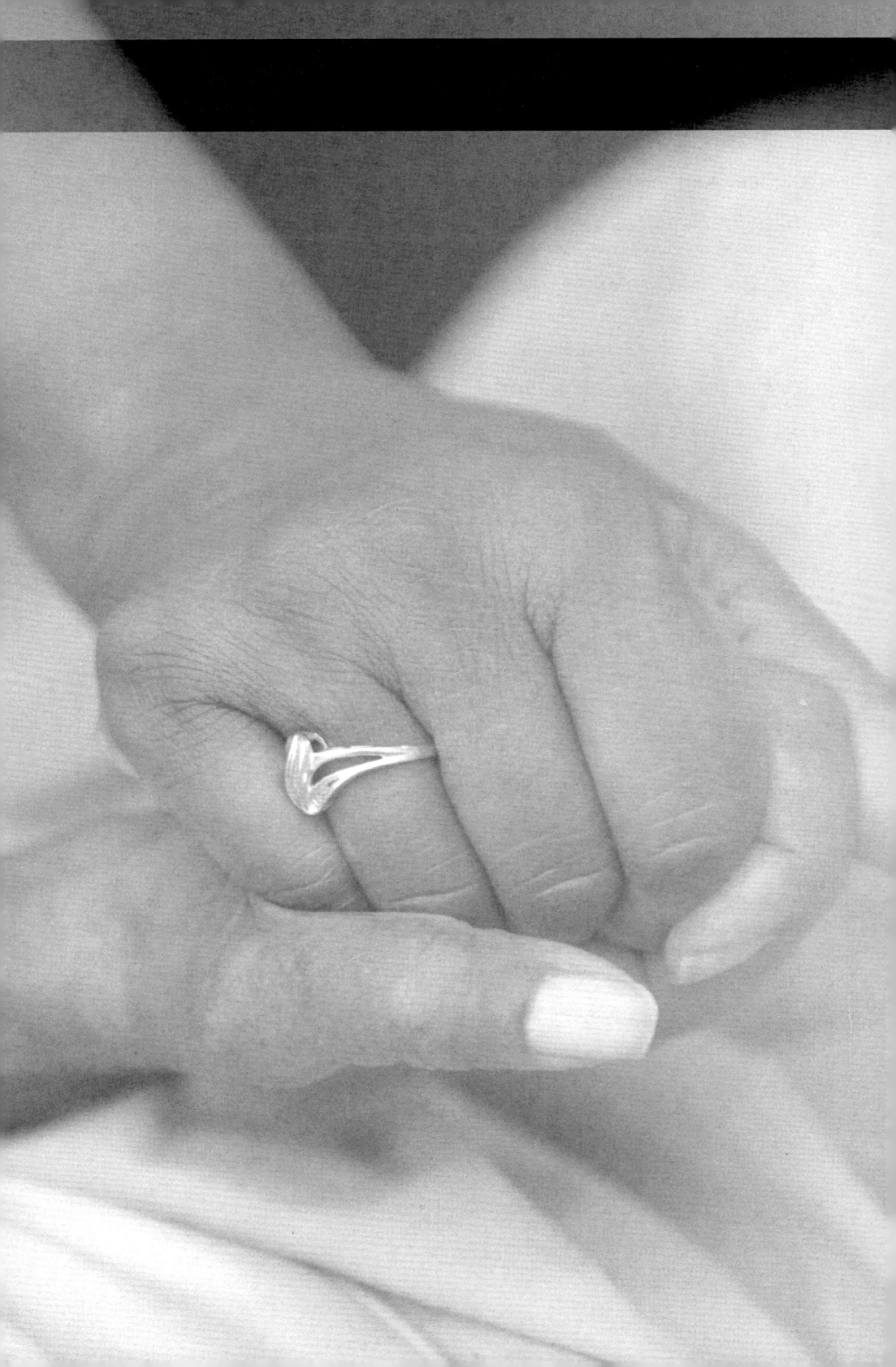

Table of Contents

Foreword — I

Chapter 1   Caregiving is the Hardest Job You'll Ever Love - Dr. Paula's Story   1

Chapter 2   Life on the Front Porch   15

Chapter 3   Advocating for Your Loved One is Required: Charles and Jeannette Ware   25

Chapter 4   Focus on What You Can Control: Diane Byrd and Mom   33

Chapter 5   Don't Take It Personal: Roberta Brown and Erica Wilson   41

Chapter 6   Learning Patience, Vigilance and Humility: Eddie, Gwen McGee, Tracy and Vivian Jackson   49

Chapter 7   Laughter is the Best Medicine: The Story of Kim Ewing and Mom Dorothy   57

Chapter 8   Sharing the Caregiving as a Family - The Story of Rosie, Inealia & Mattie's care for Mom Mabel   65

Chapter 9   One Day at a Time - The Story of Doris "Dot" Stanley   73

Chapter 10   A Man Can Take Care of His Mom - The Story of Roger Young and Mom Lillie   81

Chapter 11   Exposing the Myths: Understanding Alzheimer's and Dementia   89

Chapter 12   Now That I'm Here, What Do I Do? Where Do I Go?   105

Foreword

Dr. Paula Duren has made it her mission to provide more knowledge and support to African American caregivers. What is it about the African American experience that makes caregiving unique in this population? Why do we need more focus on African Americans? Isn't dementia a brain disorder that affects African Americans in a similar way to Non-Hispanic Whites? There are lots of reasons why we need more attention paid to caregiving in African American families. First, while older African Americans suffer higher rates of dementia than do Non-Hispanic White older adults, they are less likely to be diagnosed, and when they are diagnosed it is more likely to be in a more advanced stage of the disease. There has been a lack of attention to dementia in African Americans for a whole host of contextual reasons including bias and discrimination, a relative lack of medical providers in many African American communities, and the lack of outreach and engagement from health professionals to African Americans about recognizing the signs of dementia. Second, African American caregivers are neglected even more than those with dementia. African American caregivers typically have less knowledge about their patient's dementia and less support.

Caregiving is the most studied and discussed topic in gerontology across the past 50 years. Despite this intense focus, there has been a lack of attention to and understanding of caregiving in African Americans—particularly among adult children or other family members. On the Front Porch changes that. The stories you are about to read from caregivers offer unique lessons, as well as the hundreds of families Dr. Duren has worked with through the years. This book offers shared learnings from the African American community on caregiving; how to help your older parent or loved one while simultaneously using the experience to grow as a person through the caregiving role.

Dr. Duren masterfully weaves together a person-centered approach to assisting a person with dementia, and a positive psychology approach to embracing the caregiving role. The real-life stories that Dr. Duren shares illustrate the lessons she has learned through her own experience as a caregiver to her parents and through working with hundreds of African American caregivers herself. Dr. Duren created a training program based on the principles illustrated in her book, and the stories from actual caregivers make them come alive. On the Front Porch is a road map for African American caregivers on how to appreciate the person who has dementia, how to survive and grow during caregiving and how to use the experience to enrich one's life. Dr. Duren has gifted us with a treasure in this book.

Peter A. Lichtenberg, Ph.D., ABPP
Director Institute of Gerontology and Merrill Palmer Skillman Institute
WSU Distinguished Service Professor of Psychology
Wayne State University

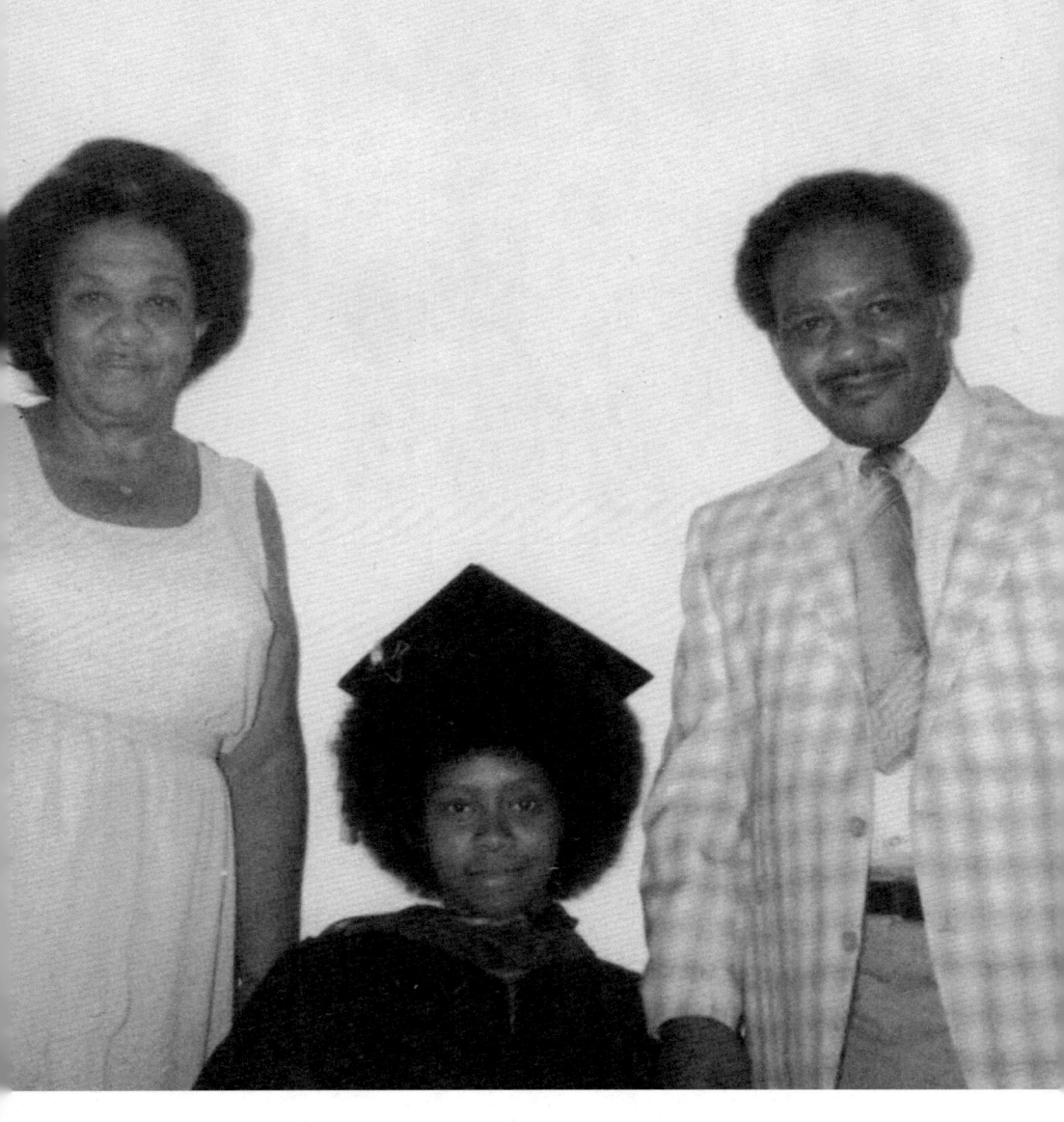

Chapter 1
Caregiving is the Hardest Job You'll Ever Love
- Dr. Paula's Story

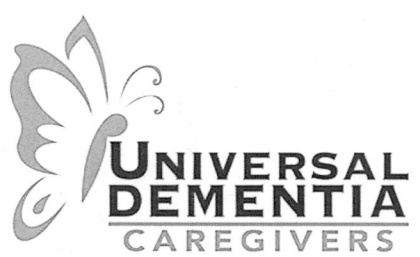

www.universaldementia.org

"We found out my dad had been diagnosed with vascular dementia when he had a car accident and that he had been taking medication for two years. It's common for people to hide It. His dementia developed much more slowly than my mom's…".- Dr. Paula Duren

The Beginning

One of the first indications that my mother had Alzheimer's was the day I got a call from a kind shopkeeper at Novi Mall, a large, popular shopping mall in Novi, Michigan, just outside Detroit. My mother lived in Ferndale, nearly 20 miles away. She had driven herself there to go shopping and forgot how to get home. God put her in that shopkeeper's hands. "Your mother is disoriented, and she really doesn't know where she is," he said. This was surprising because my mother took care of all the finances around the house and wrote all the checks. She was traditionally sharp.

> I think most families have warnings and oftentimes don't pay attention to some of the early indicators—it's not like you want to take their lives from them because they should maintain some independence as long as possible. If they start doing things like being forgetful and leaving the stove on, you need to intervene.

Weeks before the shopkeeper's call, I noticed Mom was starting to have trouble with the family bills and banking management. I began to help her, but didn't consider it a significant concern. The call to retrieve her from the mall was all the warning we needed. We started doing things to help and support her. Whenever she needed to go somewhere, somebody took her. She was very social, so she didn't mind that.

We took her to the doctor and described what happened and that was when we were told she probably had some type of dementia. I think most families have warnings and oftentimes don't pay attention to some of the early indicators—it's not like you want to take their lives from them because they should maintain their independence as long as possible. If they start doing things like being forgetful and leaving the stove on, you need to take action to protect them.

We knew this was going to advance so we put a care team around her and started thinking about what else we needed to do in the house. My mother also had rheumatoid arthritis. We did a home assessment to create the right environment that would support both Mom and Dad, and started converting the home to make it adaptable as mom's disease progressed. In the care planning process, we talked to family about what types of things she might need. At this time, dad hadn't shown symptoms yet, so we were focused on taking care of mom.

The care team included a physician, family members, and other caregivers. We also developed a communication plan with specific roles and responsibilities of various family members and what we would do to support mom and dad. Dad was still able to do for himself for a long while until he wasn't and then we had to put a full-fledged care team around them both. We knew we needed somebody to stay in the house, somebody to cook, and somebody to clean and make sure the house was safe. We put in ramps and changed out the carpeting to wood floors for mom's wheelchair. Over time, dad also needed a chair.

Too often caregivers don't know who they are serving. We never thought about putting mom or dad in a nursing facility. You need to have a real conversation regarding your loved ones wishes as they age. Some older adults desire to live forever (like my mom) and will be comfortable in a nursing facility. While others (like my dad) made it very clear he wanted to age in place at home. You should know your loved ones well enough to understand their wishes and desires.

We were committed to keeping them at home to age in place and if it ever got to a point that we couldn't, we would find a way. But we knew we could. We had constant contact with doctors and access to them, so we knew there was nothing we couldn't do at home even to the level of hospice, so we allowed them to transition at home. We've found that aging in place helped them to live longer and feel a bit more stable.

Every family must make the placement decision that works for them. People shouldn't read my story and say, "I'm going to do that." It's more than a notion. I thought I was smart. I lost part of my family because we got into a conflict and we couldn't resolve it. We did good starting out. As the disease progressed for both of them, our family conflicts got worse. What we learned later is that 25 percent of families that get into conflict never get out.

You make decisions about what you can do. If you can't keep your loved ones at home, you should consider a place that you have evaluated that will serve them properly.

I believe in honoring our loved ones with dignity. It is important to know what they would want for themselves. It's best to have that conversation while they're healthy. It's the role of the caregiver to know their desires. Sometimes we act like people with dementia aren't still alive and they are. Their spirit and soul are still in them and we need to make sure to honor them every day.

Our motto for Universal Dementia is "honor who they were, love who they are, and welcome who they become." They're going through changes affecting their behavior, but their spirit doesn't change.

Mom and Dad: Understanding Them Before Serving Them

My dad, William, was a Bishop and my mom, Sue Della was First Lady. My parents had the gift of discernment and wisdom. We were a strong, religious, traditional African American family. We were properly closed and judgmental, but it changed over time. My dad always said there's nobody better or worse than you. Mom was strong, independent, outspoken, and she could read your spirit and would say out loud what she thought you were going through.

My parents were married for over 60 years. They were almost 90 years old when they died. Mom died in 2012 and dad died 9 months later in 2013. I moved dad into my house and recreated his room in my home so he could have something familiar. He came with my brother-in-law who was the main caregiver, my sister and my nephew. My family had split at that point. I was given guardianship over my parents and there was major drama over that.

The biggest thing mom and dad did together was church. Friday night after church, we stopped at White Castle. It was a tradition. When my father would come home from work, we would sit for a traditional dinner. He would get up from the table and he would say "Sue that was good." My mom was the worst cook in the world and one day I leaned over and asked him, "Daddy, what did you just eat because I had the same thing and I don't know what it was."

"I have no idea, but it was good," he said

I knew he was just trying to keep the peace because I would have said something. Mom couldn't cook. Everything went into one pot. The only things she could make was ice cream and chicken and dumplings.

Momma was very strict and, in some ways, mean. My dad had a very quiet spirit, but he was very insightful. I would talk with him about what I learned in school about psychiatric issues and he would talk about it as the Bible would present it. That was one of the most wonderful things that I was given from my father in coming to understand people-- we are human and divine and we should learn how to manage both parts.

Dad had also been a line worker at General Motors for 35 years before he had a heart attack. Then he became a minister full-time. We spent our time traveling across the state spending weekends at different churches. Dad was a lead bishop for the Pentecostal church. He was brilliant for only having had a high school education. He could talk to an electrician, a concrete mason or a lawyer and gain immediate respect because of his knowledge of their crafts. He also helped build churches. He could talk to anybody. He was a gifted minister.

They were good parents. They did the best they could do.

Some people are so angry as adults with their parents and if you're angry at my age, let it go. Your parents did the best they could do. My job was to make sure their last days were their best days and that's how I viewed my job. It's important to give them permission to leave if they're ready to go.

I had to grow to that point. I had taken my mother to emergency for the third time in three months. We sat there all night. The emergency room was full; we had a room and no doctors came to check on us in that time frame. And I was sitting there praying and I just needed to communicate with God. "Lord, am I doing this for me or for her?" Mom was in a death cycle while transitioning. She hadn't spoken to anyone in two days. She had a collapsed lung. She was lying on the gurney, and I leaned over, and I said "Ma, I'm really sorry for putting you through this. They stick needles in you, they draw blood and that's painful for you. I'm taking you home. I don't care who walks in the door. I promise I will never make you go through this again. I won't let them poke you and prod you one more time."

In the process of me saying that to her, she opened her eyes and she said, "I love you."

She hadn't spoken in two days. That was my confirmation that I was doing the right thing. At that point, the doctor walked in and I said, "There's no need for your services. I'm taking her home." My mother died five days later. It's almost like I gave her permission to go because I stopped trying to insist that she live.

One of the greatest gifts, I think, anyone can be given is to be given permission to walk the last journey in someone's life.

Feeling Helpless and Hopeless

Parents aren't supposed to get sick. They're supposed to take care of us. Many people struggle when these roles reverse. I had an appreciation for what I thought we were. But you don't know what you're going to go through taking care of a person with a terminal illness until you do it. Like I said, I thought I was smart. The disease drove me to my knees. I prayed more. I asked for guidance.

I remember once when my mother was going through a phase; she would just sit and cry and there was nothing I could do. I tried everything. I would touch her. I tried to distract her, give her alternatives, everything short of medication and finally I came to a place of peace. I said to myself "you just need to be comfortable and be present in this moment." I just sat there, held her hand with tears running down my face until she fell off to sleep and I fell asleep. The next morning she woke up and she was fine.

There's a helplessness that comes over you, especially when they cry and they're so angry and they're just lashing out at you. Many caregivers struggle with this. You're doing everything you know how to do and they're just cussing you out, saying you don't love them and that you're stealing their money and you aren't doing anything for them. "I hate you," and "get out of my room."

If the emotional expressions are affecting you, go outside and breathe; call and talk to somebody; walk around a bit. If there is any nice thing about dementia – if there is a nice thing – it's that they soon forget. They may forget the incident, but they don't forget the emotion. It's about how you the caregiver can be a comfort to someone who is losing their own mental capacity while being kind to yourself.

That's why I always wanted the interaction to be positive. I was kind, I was humble. I was supportive. They remember the emotional connection. I only wanted people with good energy around my parents. My job was to keep the environment positive and calm.

Dad's disease progressed slower than mom's. My mom's Alzheimer's progressed quickly. I remember lying in bed with dad to tell him that mom had passed. It was probably one of the hardest things I had ever done. He still had capacity. He called her Sue. Dad would say "where's Sue?" I had to tell him that mom died, and he became silent. He knew what I was saying even though he had diminished capacity. There was a debate about whether he should go to the funeral, but I know he needed that psychological closure. He did good after that.

Nearing the End

I ran from my house to their house every day. I was worn down even though dad had someone with him all the time. Then conflict started happening in the family and there were major disruptions with siblings and nieces and nephews, and I had to go back to the judge to get control over the house. I had to make it like a nursing home and create a schedule with visiting hours. My family didn't like the changes. It caused more confusion; eventually, we had to stop visitation. It was tough. It isn't like you walk away having lost half of your family and don't feel it.

God has a way of working things out. Family is not necessarily who you were born with. I tell caregivers that sometimes you find a new family for support. You can't change grown people. Stop expecting people to do something when you know they won't. You need to free them and yourself – start the healing process.

My professional training as a psychologist helped me cognitively because I knew what to expect. But knowing what to expect and living it are two different things. I could explain the process to my family and the caregivers. But you don't really understand until it hits you personally. I could anticipate what to expect so in that respect my academic background was helpful. Many caregivers hope their loved ones will get better. I always prayed, let your will be done. Strengthen us to give the needed support.

Self-care is essential. I went and exercised every day to do what I had to do to stay healthy. Many caregivers don't see themselves as a priority. I was journaling daily. I write a lot. I'm really an introvert even though many people don't believe that about me.

The Birthing of Universal Dementia

I'm a believer that sometimes God takes you through things for yourself and sometimes He takes us through things for other people. This caregivers program was birthed out of my pain, struggles and experiences.

I used journaling as an emotional outlet. Journaling became my way of coping. I was angry, sad, pathetic, excited, sad and happy…you name any emotion and it was in this journal. I did not know I was actually outlining a tool to help other caregivers.

One night I asked God to show me what to do with this journal. When I went to bed I was awakened in the middle of the night. I grabbed my ink pen and he gave me the title of a program containing seven care strategies. These strategies are designed to empower caregivers to effectively support their loved one spiritually, physically and emotionally. This proven approach has been recognized as an evidence-based program and was published as such in the Clinical Gerontologist Journal, 2022.

Today through my nonprofit Universal Dementia Caregivers, we offer Lunch & Learn Bootcamps, exercise classes, training programs, support groups and the very popular caregivers boot camp full day empowerment sessions. The foundation for all of this came from mom and dad. That's why I'm so passionate about this work.

I focus on caring for the caregiver. I chose to focus on the African American caregiver because:

1. The prevalence of dementia is higher in communities of color.

2. We're oftentimes the last ones to get a diagnosis.

3. We need to educate earlier to get people to start planning earlier, before it's too late for medication to work.

4. We are less likely to reach out to the medical community because of mistrust. (Our history fuels this mistrust because of how we've been mistreated.)

5. It has been shown that black people are less likely to be referred to a specialist. I want black people to insist on being referred to a neurologist. You have a voice and you need to learn how to use it.

Mom's sassiness and dad's personal insight and kindness are probably a combination of who I am. I believe in fighting for the underdog which is what I'm doing with our newly formed non-profit. Universal Dementia Caregivers. I'm always trying to figure out how we help the person who is incapable of helping themselves. That's where I find myself now. We are tiny compared to others, but we make a difference and we want you to know that we see you, we really see you. We want to be part of your solution, and give you permission to hurt.

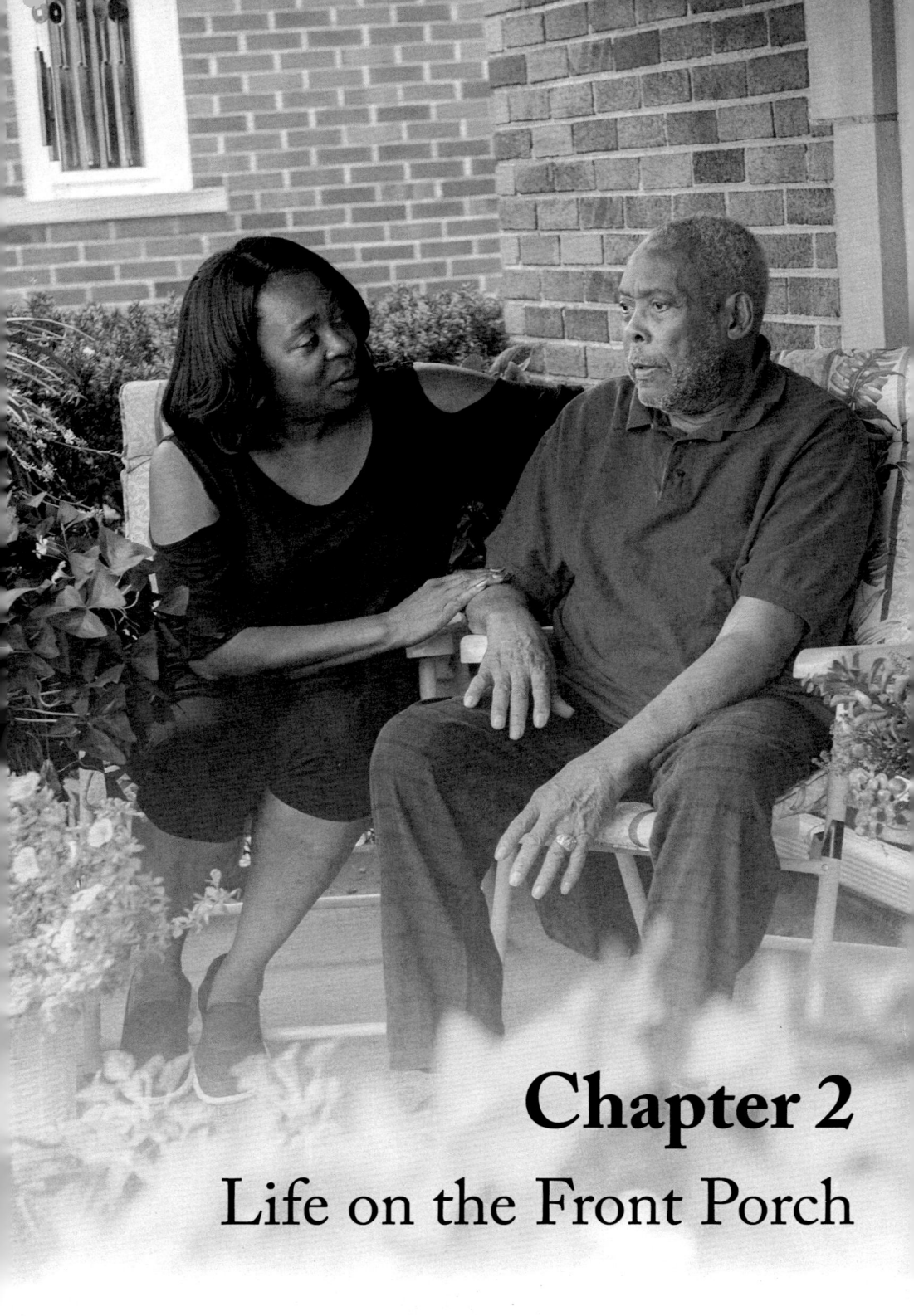

Chapter 2
Life on the Front Porch

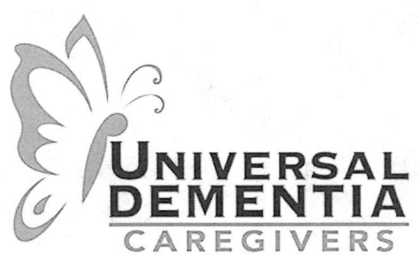

www.universaldementia.org

After a long day, African American families retired to the front porch to sip cool drinks, talk, and welcome visitors. They brought out banjos, metal tubs, and later radios and record players to sing songs and tell stories. Women snapped homegrown green beans into aprons on their laps, braided each other's hair or shared coffee and pound cake. Couples sometimes had their first dates on the front porch, under the night sky and dreamed about what life might be like without the weight of oppression and poverty.

The front porch has played such an integral part of the African American experience that it was included in the design of the National Museum of African American History and Culture in Washington, DC. The museum has a "Porch", the large covered area visitors pass through to reach the museum's south-facing entrance. The architects designed one for this museum to reference the historical and cultural uses of porches throughout the African Diaspora. At Howard University in Washington, D.C. an area called "The Porch" is the hub today for student life.

Michael Dolan, author of **The American Porch: An Informal History of an Informal Place** says the origin of the front porch can be traced to several countries, including Italy, Spain, India and Africa—having brought those traditions to America as part of the great melting pot. Enslaved Africans were the first in America to universally build houses with porches.

Germane Barnes, a lecturer at the University of Miami School of Architecture refers to the porch as a "sacred stoop". "It was a place that allowed you to do things in your own home without costing you. It was also not completely private as it was outside, where the police could still accost you or random individuals could berate you with racial slurs," said Barnes.

With all this rich history in mind, I titled this exploration into the lives of African American caregivers facing the challenges of tending to their loved ones and how they are coping with the changes brought on by dementia and Alzheimer's disease: **On the Front Porch**.

Conversations of Resilience & Devotion

In my conversations with these families, I found resilience, devotion, and coping mechanisms that should inspire and educate us all on the unique position that many of these caregivers find themselves in. All family caregivers need support and resources, but African American caregivers experience increased challenges and deserve special recognition. I know firsthand the demands brought on by the deterioration of the brain because both of my parents suffered from the debilitating effects of dementia-related diseases. Mom lived with Alzheimer's and dad dealt with vascular dementia.

> My purpose for writing this book is to show the extraordinary strength and resilience of African American caregivers who are often overlooked and overworked in their sacrifice.

My purpose for writing this book is to show the extraordinary strength and resilience of African American caregivers who are often overlooked and overworked in their sacrifice. From a cultural standpoint, many of the older adults suffering from these diseases imparted much of their wisdom while sitting **On the Front Porch**. African Americans born and raised all over the country remember summers spent with grandmothers, aunts, and neighbors sharing stories while watching over children playing in the yard. And now the torch has been passed to us to share that wisdom with the next generation who will care for the most vulnerable and prized members of our families.

My hope is to create greater awareness for caregivers who face tough decisions every day and to provide information on resources available to help meet their needs and those of their loved ones.

Safe & Secure on the Porch

The front porch played an important, historical role in African American culture in America. It was where we ate popsicles, drank sweet tea, and listened to the heavy sound of crickets as we watched "lightning bugs" flicker and float through the air. The porch was more than a simple structure for rocking chairs and airing out rugs. It was our safe space during the era of Jim Crow laws, which enforced racial segregation.

The porch was where we learned about our black identity and

where we laughed listening to "grown folk business" and the latest neighborhood gossip. It was our refuge, a place for healing and a place where little black girls and boys played, danced, and laughed under the watchful eyes of family and neighbors. We were often relegated to "staying on the porch" so as not to get in any trouble.

In cities like Detroit, Atlanta and even Washington, D.C., the porch became a classroom, a barbershop or depending on the community's needs, a place to pass down wisdom and share family care expectations for our elders. On Sundays, the front porch was an extension of the church. Thus, caregiving is often rooted in a strong reliance on faith and respect.

Suffering in Silence

Traditionally, African Americans have kept health issues at home because of a lack of trust of white healthcare professionals and institutions. Due to less-than-ideal conditions at some nursing facilities, relatives were kept at home so they could be treated with dignity. The front porch was a safe place to share stories about the family illnesses, especially when family secrets remained hidden, including what happened to "crazy Uncle Joe" who was kept in the back room for years -- I believe he may have been living with a dementia disease. It is still believed by many that dementia is a mental illness and not a brain disease. Thus, there is a tendency to hide dementia-related diseases.

A recent policy paper by the Alzheimer's Association noted: "Alzheimer's disease has been identified as an emerging public health crisis among African American communities. This silent epidemic of Alzheimer's has slowly invaded the African American community and will continue to grow as numbers of African American baby boomers enter the age of risk where they are also more likely to need care as they age due to higher rates of chronic illnesses such as diabetes, hypertension, and high cholesterol."

Many of those "baby boomers" (born between 1946 and 1964) are the generation now either suffering from dementia diseases and Alzheimer's or they are "sandwiched" between caring for an older person and a younger person under age 18 or caring for more than one older person. It has been suggested that "many people will spend more of their time and resources caring for their aging parents than they did raising their own children."[1]

> Many people will spend more of their time and resources caring for their aging parents than they did raising their own children.

A God-given Responsibility

These type of caregivers are less likely to ask for support. They spend a significant amount of their hard-earned money and devote more of their time caring for loved ones, without the assistance of paid in-home care. Caring for a loved one is often considered a responsibility

---

1. Barry Jacobs, clinical psychologist, wrote "the culture that shapes us frames our perceptions of the sacrifices we make and the meanings we derive. African Americans may cope with caregiving better because their culture enables them to feel more positively about it."

and not a burden. African Americans may experience less burden because the caregiver role is often viewed as their God-given responsibility.

Much of this responsibility comes historically from religious teaching where to this day churches maintain a sick and shut-in list of members who are cared for by a body of believers. They support the family by dropping off meals, praying with the caregiver, running errands, or doing minor chores to help lighten the load.

> 57% of African American caregivers spend more time caregiving on average, spending 30 hours per week caring for their loved one. That's compared to 33 percent of white caregivers, who averaged 20 hours per week.
>
> ~ Alzheimer's Association's 2015 Alzheimer's Disease Facts and Figures.

According to the AARP/NAC, many African American caregivers feel they have no choice in the matter and so the responsibility to support one another just kicks in naturally. A "majority find a sense of purpose" in caregiving — more than among white caregivers. That sense of purpose could be defined in religious terms ("doing God's will") or family terms ("giving back to someone who took good care of me").

African American Caregiving: A Unique Experience

Caregiving is a sign of appreciation for our elders. It is during these times that siblings and cousins pull together to take care of mom and dad. There is typically no differentiation between parents, aunts, and uncles because "of the village." Often, several generations of families live under the same roof so it is natural that the care of grandma and grandpa would occur in the home as they age. Even though family structures are changing, caring for loved ones in the home appears to continue as a shared value in our communities.

This legacy of love has resulted in an ongoing devotion that's been passed down from one family to another. The example that's been set remains a unique characteristic of the African American family which is statistically different from others:

- 57% of African American caregivers spend more time caregiving on average, spending 30 hours per week caring for their loved one. That's compared to 33 percent of white caregivers, who averaged 20 hours per week, according to the Alzheimer's Association's 2015 Alzheimer's Disease Facts and Figures. [1]

- While African American caregivers spend similar amounts of money as white caregivers, their financial burden is higher due to lower average household incomes. African American caregivers devote more than 34 percent of their annual income to expenses associated with providing care, compared with 14 percent for white caregivers.[1]

- African American caregivers tend to be younger (42.7 years

---

1. Barry Jacobs, clinical psychologist, wrote "the culture that shapes us frames our perceptions of the sacrifices we make and the meanings we derive. African Americans may cope with caregiving better because their culture enables them to feel more positively about it."

old) than white caregivers (52.5 years old), according to the National Alliance for Caregiving and AARP's 2015 Caregiving in the U.S. survey.[1]

- The disease is more prevalent among African Americans than among Caucasians – with estimates ranging from 14 percent to almost 100 percent higher. The number of African Americans at risk for Alzheimers at age 65 or older is expected to more than double to 6.9 million by 2030.[1]

As we continue to explore the importance of these familial ties and what they mean to the caregiving experience for African Americans, you will hopefully gain some takeaways that will not only touch your heart but will also provide insights that will help you navigate the legal, financial and emotional challenges that come with caring for loved ones living with dementia related diseases. This glimpse into the homes of these African American caregivers is an important step to understanding their caregiving experiences.

---

1. Barry Jacobs, clinical psychologist, wrote "the culture that shapes us frames our perceptions of the sacrifices we make and the meanings we derive. African Americans may cope with caregiving better because their culture enables them to feel more positively about it."

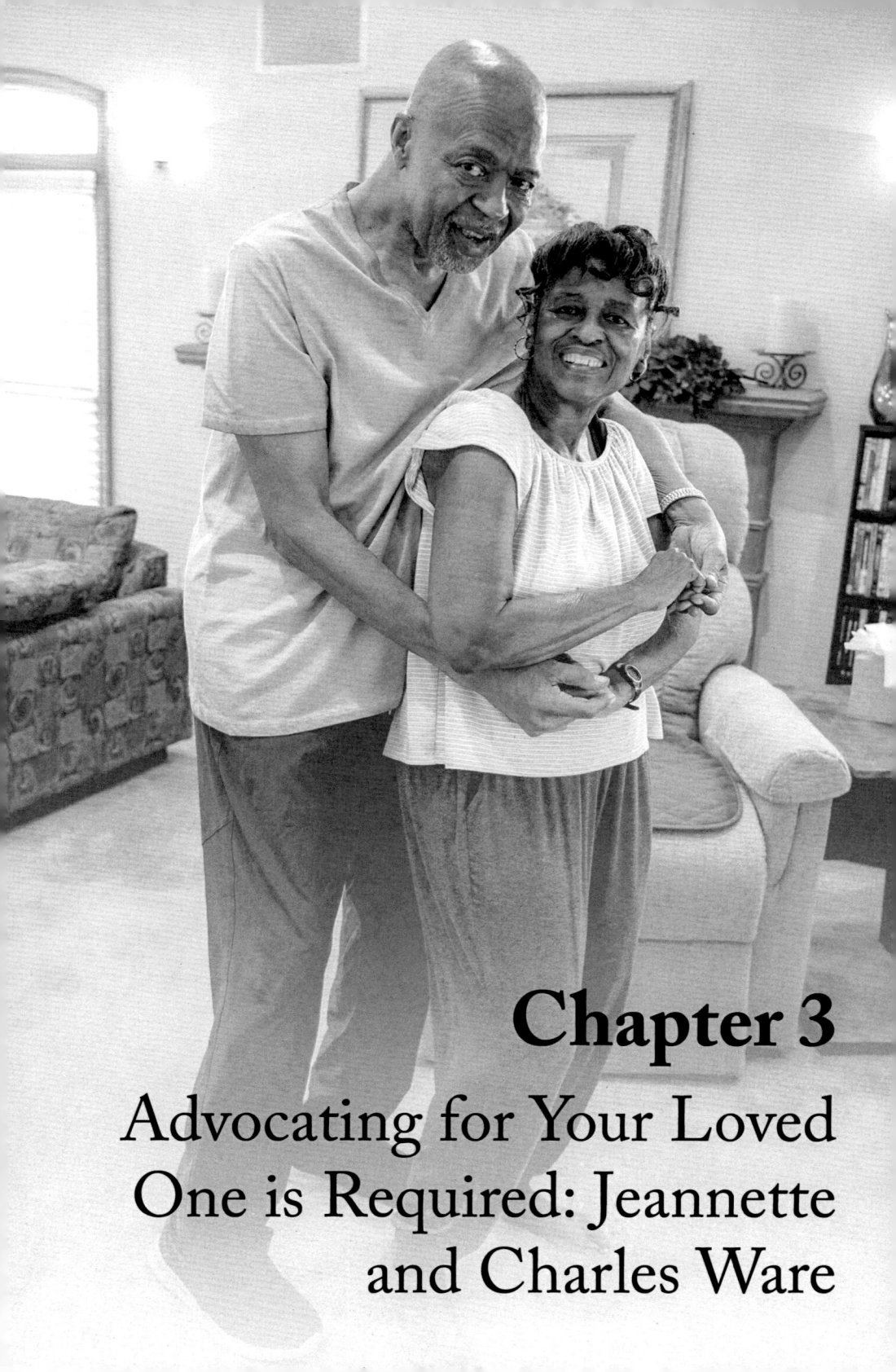

Chapter 3
Advocating for Your Loved One is Required: Jeannette and Charles Ware

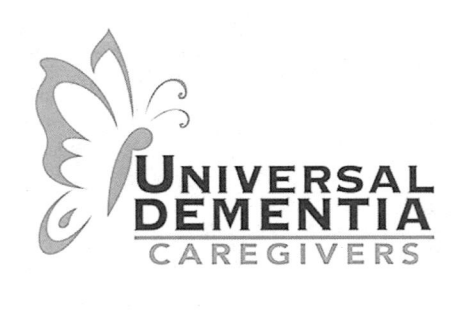

UNIVERSAL DEMENTIA CAREGIVERS

www.universaldementia.org

Meet Jeanette and Charles Ware

For four years Jeanette Ware pushed for a proper diagnosis with four different neurologists. Test after test, over and over she was told that her husband's confusion was due to sleep apnea. Finally, "someone really listened and talked to us."

Life Before Dementia

When Jeanette and Charles Ware were building their dream house in Detroit's Victoria Park, no detail was too small for Charles, an Air Force veteran who worked in the electronics department at General Motors until he retired in 2017.

Charles was a take charge man, detailed-oriented man. During the home build out, he took pride in overseeing each task.

"We were a headache," says Jeanette, recalling with a laugh how the builder kept saying, "We don't do it that way!"

By the time the house was done in 1994, the builder couldn't get away from the couple fast enough. Charles put his footprint and special touch everywhere throughout the house, from paint colors to light fixtures. He researched everything from A to Z, even down to his clothes. He would travel as far as New York City to shop for the latest fashion and the perfect suit. He liked things that were unique.

Accepting A New Normal

Things are different now. First, he began forgetting things that Jeanette knew were familiar to him. One day, she asked him to count for her and he didn't know what number came after 99. She started testing him more; she didn't like the results. "I had to make sure the evidence I was seeing was really happening," she said.

In 2020, Charles was diagnosed with dementia and Parkinson's disease. Jeanette, a former flight attendant and bank loan authorizer who later worked for herself selling insurance, became a fierce advocate for her husband.

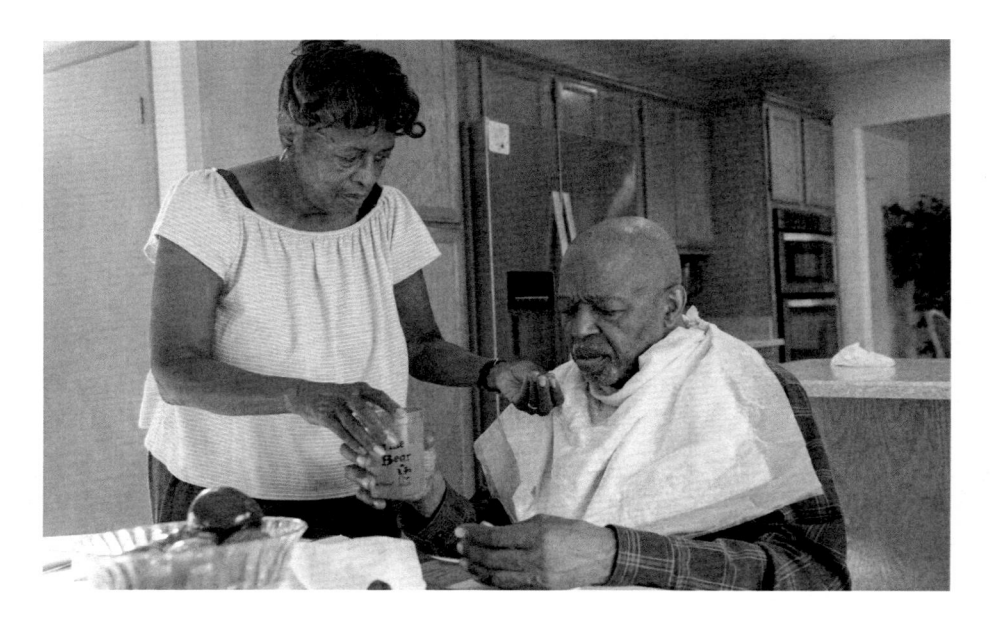

Much has changed for the couple, both 74, who've known each other since they were students at Central High School in Detroit. Charles, who now goes to daycare, is like a child who needs Jeanette to get his shoes on, she says. "I have to make sure he goes to bed and goes to the bathroom. If we go to the store, I have to watch him."

It's not easy. "I've done a lot of crying the last couple months," Jeanette shares. "I have good days and bad days. Charles has good and bad days," she says. "This is what it is. I cannot change it. I just do a lot of praying."

Jeanette cooks the meals and manages the finances. Their home now has grab bars in the bathrooms and an extra rail to go upstairs, special chairs for Charles and a walker he doesn't like to use. Jeanette tries not to let him walk alone.

Today the couple sit at the table in their tidy kitchen surrounded by warm golden walls and photos of their two daughters nearby. Their roles have changed. Jeanette does most of the talking now, although Charles was always "the talker." He chimes in once in a while, prompted by her chatter. His voice soft and measured.

The signs were there. Charles was religious about getting his annual PSA test for prostate cancer. When Jeanette reminded him, he said, "I don't know what that is." He then started struggling and stumbling when they practiced ballroom dancing together. "He couldn't get the steps if they threw something new in there. It was like a puzzle."

Finding Joy in the Little Things

And she's learning, even from Charles. He recently had a stumble and found himself on the floor. "I couldn't get him up," says Jeanette, who decided to let him sit there for a while as she finished up a task. "The next thing I know, he got up. I noticed if you let them do what they need to do, they will do it. But if you're helping 24/7, they won't do it because they're relying on you." The lesson: "Let them be free to do what they can physically do." She's also learning to recognize his limitations. " I have to slow up and be more patient and not get upset because I can get upset," she says.

> As for looking ahead, Jeanette chooses to take things one day at a time. "I just have to live in the moment and understand that this is new," she says.

The couple lost a daughter in 2005 from complications related to breast cancer. They get a lot of support from their nieces who regularly check on them. "They are a blessing," she says. "We do group texts and we pray; they know what I'm going through." In the meantime, this journey is teaching Jeanette a lot about herself and how she looks at life now, she says. "I do have the strength, the ability to deal with some things I never thought I'd have to."

And she's discovering joy in small things, like making breakfast for Charles; seeing how much he appreciates it. "I'll say, 'I love you,' and he'll say, 'I love you more.' And he'll hold my hand and still to this day he'll open the door for me knowing I should go first."

Charles, who loves to listen to music, especially jazz, still dances with Jeanette. That was the one thing this tall, soft-spoken man and loving husband said about himself, "I always was a dancer and I said I'm not giving it up."

As for looking ahead, Jeanette chooses to take things one day at a time. "I just have to live in the moment and understand that this is new," she says. "This is something new. He was my husband, he took care of me and now I have to take care of him. I miss the intimacy. We're no longer intimate."

DR. PAULA'S INSIGHTS:

After reading **Jeanette and Charles Ware's** story, I want you to note the following key takeaways:

1. **Your role will change.** You might be the wife, daughter, son or husband, but you need to be prepared to accept your changing role as a caregiver. This will require time to accept these adjustments. Living without the intimacy that was an important part of your relationship is difficult for couples who had sexually active lives. You learn to value little moments of intimacy – remembering your name; a touch or simple glance of recognition. The roles of your life will change dramatically. But Jeanette remembers: Charles is the same person. He's just at a different place in life. She had to change and be more patient.

2. **You are the advocate.** As a caregiver, you need to understand that you are the advocate, and you must insist on being part of the care planning process. You must accept the changes that are happening to your loved one because you become even more important in the life of your loved one, and you help other people respect and honor them.

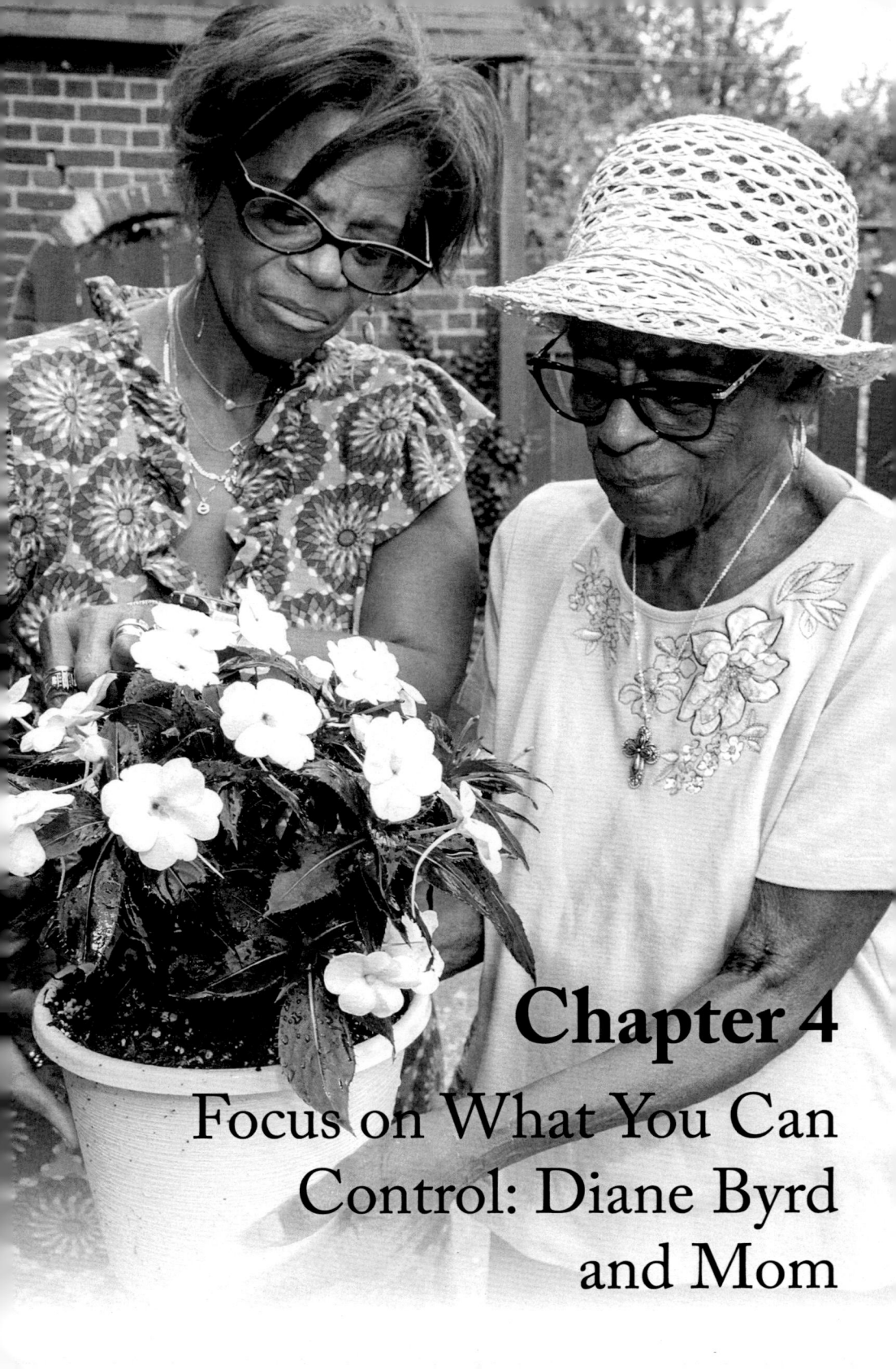

Chapter 4
Focus on What You Can Control: Diane Byrd and Mom

UNIVERSAL DEMENTIA CAREGIVERS

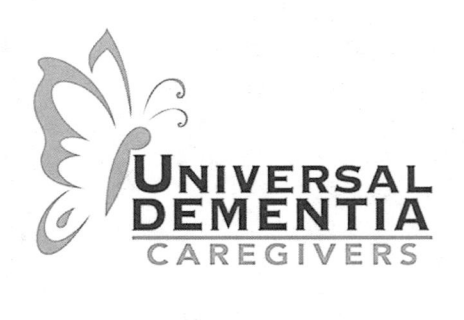

www.universaldementia.org

Meet Diane Byrd and Lois Cole

Lois Cole is surrounded by family — literally.

Four daughters and a grandson sat on either side of her one sunny September afternoon in daughter Diane Byrd's Detroit living room. They have been the core of the 93-year-old matriarch's caregiving team since she was diagnosed with dementia in 2015.

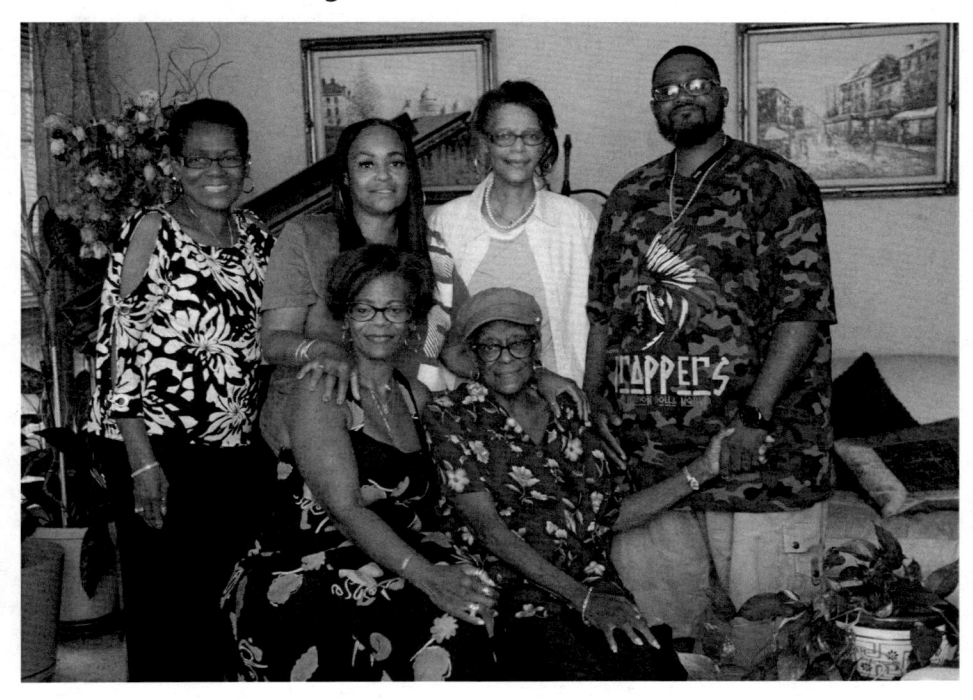

Resentment, Hurt Feelings and Disagreements

Diane brought her mother in her home to live with her more than 30 years ago after Lois' husband died. At that time Lois was sharing her home with the youngest daughter, Mary, 49, and her three kids. This living arrangement was overwhelming for Lois.

For Lois, who raised 10 children and many grandchildren, staying with Diane means a smooth transition as she ages in place. Diane's adjustment as primary caregiver, however, hasn't been so easy. At first, she shouldered the burden of care and began to resent her siblings for not doing more. Whenever anyone made a suggestion or questioned something, Diane got defensive.

The family seemed always to be in conflict. "I admit it was probably mostly me," she says. "I would complain: 'Nobody is doing anything.' I was stressing myself out. No one could come by without something happening. My mother probably felt that. And I didn't want to bring that on her," Diane admitted.

You Have Not Because You Ask Not

Diane, 65, has learned much about caring for someone with dementia since that time. One of the biggest lessons was learning to ask for support. "I thought it should be natural. This is their mother, too," she said. "But once I asked for help, like, 'Can you drop mom off?' That simple request helped a lot." She's grateful today for the progress the family has made. "We're finally getting to the point where we can communicate and understand that it's all for mom." As for her personal growth, she realizes she cannot change people. "I can only deal with myself. If something happens that's not to my liking, move on. Don't linger on it." Diane said. "It's a lesson other family members

> Diane advises other caregivers to learn as much as they can about dementia because everyone's loved one is different.

still struggle with, especially when it comes to a couple of siblings who don't visit or participate as the rest of us feel they should."

Sister Patricia Williams, 70, who steps in when Diane leaves town, still can't understand having to ask for help when the siblings are all in the same area. She chokes up as she wonders aloud how it can be that they all grew up in the same home, with a mother who was always there for them, one big family who didn't have much but at least had her, she says. "I want them to be here for her now. How can one mother take care of 10 kids and 10 kids can't take care of one mother?"

Still, Diane, who retired from her job doing community outreach in 2017 to spend more time at home, is thankful they've come as far as they have. "We are really, really blessed. I've seen other people dealing with it and it's one hundred times worse. Some people don't have siblings to help them. They're all by themselves."

Dementia Is Not A One Size Fits All Disease

Diane advises other caregivers to learn as much as they can about dementia because everyone's loved one is different. But perhaps, more importantly, she says: "Take care of yourself. That was my biggest fear. If I get sick, who's going to take care of us?" Realizing the importance of her own self-care motivated Diane to make peace with her siblings, something Patricia's son Adrian Cole, 46, echoes in his advice: "Y'all gotta be on the same page, because one person can't do everything."

These days, Diane accepts that not everyone can be a caregiver for someone with dementia. "I had in my mind: It's 10 of us, or however many of us, if everybody would just take a day. But it never happened," she says. "So, you just have to move on."

Moving on has allowed the siblings to enjoy their mother more. They share memories growing up in the house where everyone wanted to hang out. Lois, who worked at Hudson's department store in downtown Detroit and a Hallmark store once her older kids could take care of the younger ones, always had a project going. If she wasn't drawing or making them clothes, playing the guitar, or knitting baby blankets for the grandchildren, she was baking cookies or sweet potato pies. She'd do puzzles with them and plan picnics. One of their favorite memories is when she made Cabbage Patch dolls — not just for family but neighborhood kids, too. "I always thought she could have been a teacher," Diane recalls.

She also remembers her mother's early signs of dementia. Lois had gone to visit Diane's sister Sandra Boyd, 61, but returned saying no one was home. When Sandra called to say their mother never showed up, Diane said it was scary. "I realized she went to the wrong house." There were other clues, too, like how Lois started to struggle to understand monetary denominations when shopping.

Despite the limitations she lives with today, Lois has a fair amount of independence. "She can do a lot on her own but needs assistance," says Sandra, who tries to honor those abilities. "Whatever she can do on her own, we should let her do it."

While Diane helps with bathing and reminds her to take her pills, puts out her clothes and prepares meals, Lois dresses and feeds herself. Mealtime is one thing no one needs to remind Lois about. "She knows when it's time to eat," says Diane. If breakfast is not on the table by eight o'clock, Lois will say: "Okay, are we eating today?" The siblings laugh. She also enjoys watching television, eating out, and sitting in the yard. "She's out every day," says Diane. "It's like: Are we going out today? Are we going to get some air?"

As much as Diane and her sisters have learned along the way, it's still work being a caregiver. "No one prepares you for what it's like to have a loved one with dementia. I'm sure people look in and think you're doing a great job and everyone's happy. But it's a lot." The hardest times are when Lois gets depressed and cries. "That gets me. I don't have any control to make it better." What's also tough is when she doesn't know who I am."

Still, this journey has enriched their lives. "You become more humble and thankful," says Patricia. Sandra agrees: "You can't take anything for granted."

For Diane, she's content with her role these days. She was always taking care of somebody, including one sister who died from cancer. "I think I realized that's just my nature and that's just an assignment I've been given from God."

DR. PAULA'S INSIGHTS:

After reading **Diane Byrd and her mom Lois Cole's** story, I want you to note the following key takeaways:

1. **Your family cannot read your mind.** Learn how to ask for what you want and what you need in terms of being a caregiver. Allowing anger and resentment to build inside of you only causes more stress.

2. **Families have conflict.** This is normal and expected. You must understand that everyone experiences the loss of a loved one in different ways. It is important to learn as much as you can learn and understand where your loved one is on the dementia journey.

3. **Divine Assignment.** Embrace that caregiving for your loved one is an assignment given by God.

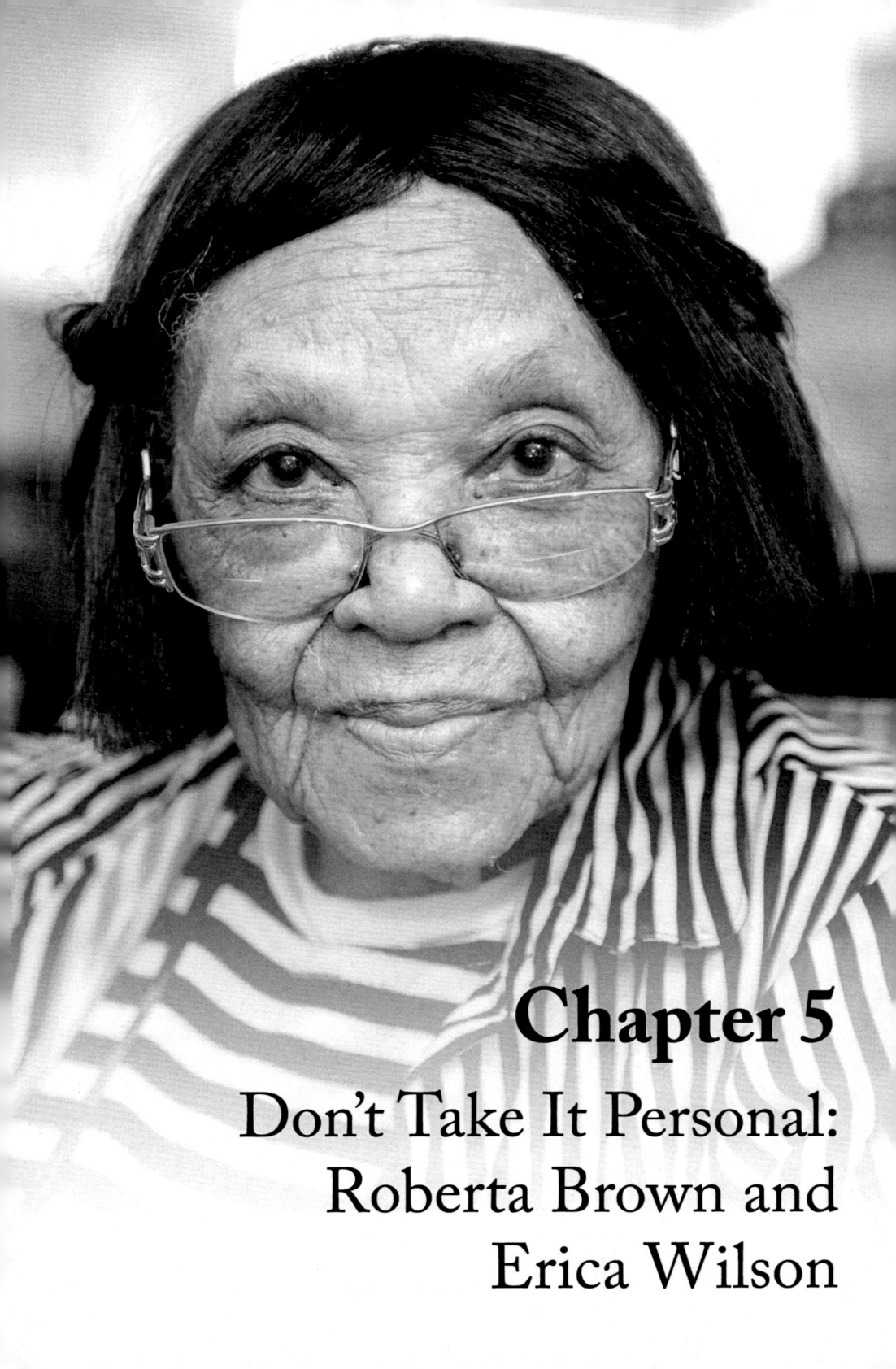

Chapter 5
Don't Take It Personal: Roberta Brown and Erica Wilson

UNIVERSAL
DEMENTIA
CAREGIVERS

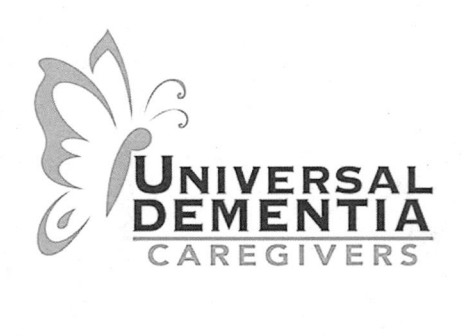

www.universaldementia.org

Meet Roberta Brown and Erica Wilson

Erica Wilson wasn't the one called upon to do much caregiving in her family. At age 52, married with no children, she was not even the assigned caregiver for her 81-year-old mother with late-stage Alzheimer's disease who is in the care of her Atlanta-based sister and only sibling.

So, when her maternal grandmother, 101-year-old Roberta Brown, needed support. She reluctantly stepped up, agreeing to move her from Georgia to Detroit.

It was not an easy decision considering her "Nana," who suffers from Alzheimer's disease, was always a bit difficult. "If you offer her steak she'll say, 'I'd rather have liver' because she usually wants the opposite of what you have."

Cherished Memories Help Create Understanding

If Roberta can be tough, Erica reminds herself she had a tough upbringing. She grew up so poor she and her siblings were separated and sent to live with other family members. "She's been working her whole life."

As a child, when Erica would visit her grandparents, she recalls feeling loved and cared for by Roberta. When she was about 12, Roberta would let her try her Yves Saint Laurent designer perfume or encourage her to polish her nails. She instructed her on which slip went with which dress and what shoes to wear. "It was exciting to have someone want to dress me up and make me pretty."

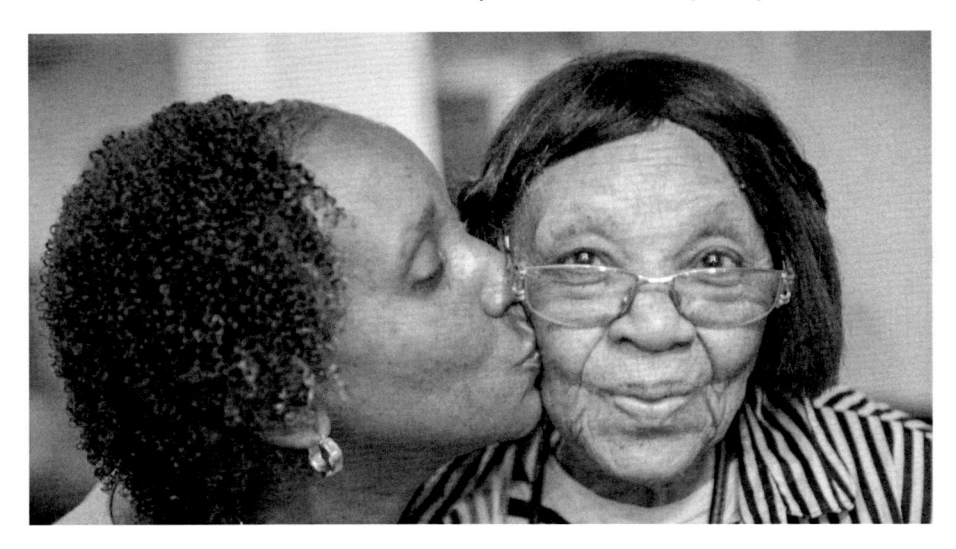

It was also around that time Erica recalls a tender memory she holds on to today–learning to French braid on Roberta's hair. "She loved for me to massage her scalp," she says. The memory is bittersweet because Roberta got one of the first perms which caused her to lose a lot of hair, says Erica. "That's why she wears wigs. She's got a spoonful of hair." Now Erica wants to make Roberta look pretty. Last year she bought her a wig to replace one she's had for years which, Erica jokes, "looked like a beaver that got into a fight."

When Roberta fussed that the new wig didn't look right, Erica styled it. "I said, 'look how beautiful you look' and she replied, 'Yes, I do.'" Erica laughs. "She doesn't wear it much but when she does, she's like Tina Turner."

Erica cherishes moments like that and is finding ways to create more memories. "Before COVID, I'd always give her a hug and kiss and she'd always be like that box right there. So one day I said, 'You give me a kiss.' And she did. Right on my cheek. And she smiled," she says. "I'm just looking for moments that she can hold on to. It's not about me."

The Decision to Find a Facility for Care

After discussing things with her husband, who manages care for both his mother and an elderly uncle, Erica decided Roberta would have to live full-time in a facility.

After months of research, Erica, settled on a bright, cheery-looking care center in Southfield, Michigan 10 miles from her home. Knowing almost no place would make her Nana happy. Erica shared, "I knew that I was going to have to do a dance," she says.

Indeed, moving in was an emotional first day for Roberta following a 10-hour drive from Georgia to Michigan "She cried like a baby," says Erica, who cried right along with her. "I didn't know what to do. But we got her in the door. Once she saw the familiarity of her furniture, that was comforting." Erica stayed with her the first few nights to ease the transition.

In many ways, she's still trying to do that as she supports Roberta while finding her way in this journey. Erica strives to be a good caregiver. She visits Roberta three days a week, does her laundry, cleans her apartment, and brings her favorite fast foods. Lately, that's Popeyes Chicken.

Without children and only being "mom" to her German Shepherd dog, who exudes sweetness and a desire to please, Erica found it difficult early on to accept that she could never truly make her grandmother happy. She could only do her best to meet her needs. In all of that, she does have one regret. "I wish I had pushed myself harder as far as getting her to the eye doctor," she says of Roberta's many missed glaucoma injections because she'd refuse to go.

Erica reminds herself to have some grace. "The biggest lesson is to give as much as you can. And on the way out the door, say, 'I did a good job. I did the best that I can. I'll see you tomorrow.' And leave it there."

> But as Erica knows, especially caring for someone with dementia, you can't take anything personally. Her advice to herself, "Forgive them and forgive yourself and put yourself in their shoes."

Erica strives to give Roberta grace, too. She recalls how Roberta owned two Chicago dry cleaning businesses in the late 1950s and early 1960s with her husband, who died about 30 years ago. Erica marvels that when her grandfather got sick, Roberta managed the business and did all the books herself. She was meticulous with bills.

She also maintained a ten-room house and a garden. Even today, Erica boasts that Roberta has read the entire Medicare book. "I think she has a high school education," Erica says. "She's smart."

Still, it's challenging as Roberta's dementia progresses. She talks regularly of moving back to Chicago and having Erica's mother care for her. And she's increasingly angry, something Erica often gets the brunt of. "She told me I never did anything for her the other day," she says. But as Erica knows, especially caring for someone with dementia, you can't take anything personally. Her advice to herself, "Forgive them and forgive yourself and put yourself in their shoes."

As for self-care? It's been tough. Erica left her job working with young children because of the pandemic and has flown to Georgia multiple times to support her younger sister with her mom.

While she tries to exercise and meditate, she finds inspirational talks by Les Brown, Iyanla Vanzant and Wayne Dyer on YouTube most helpful. She's also grateful for her caregiver support group where she can vent if she needs to. "People are wearing the same shoes," she says. "You feel like you're by yourself, but you quickly find out you're not."

Mostly, she says, she's learning to trust herself. "We are all just people trying to figure it out."

DR. PAULA'S INSIGHTS:

After reading **Erica Wilson** and her grandmother Roberta's story, I want you to note the following key takeaways I see.

1. **Forgiveness is Essential.** Forgive them and forgive yourself.

2. **Follow Peace.** It is important to learn to trust yourself. You are one human doing the best you can to care for another human. It is okay to lean into what you believe is right in those difficult moments.

3. **Location does not determine love.** Placement of a loved one in a facility is a challenge but you must make the best decision based on the information available. If the best care can't be given at home, you must find other alternatives.

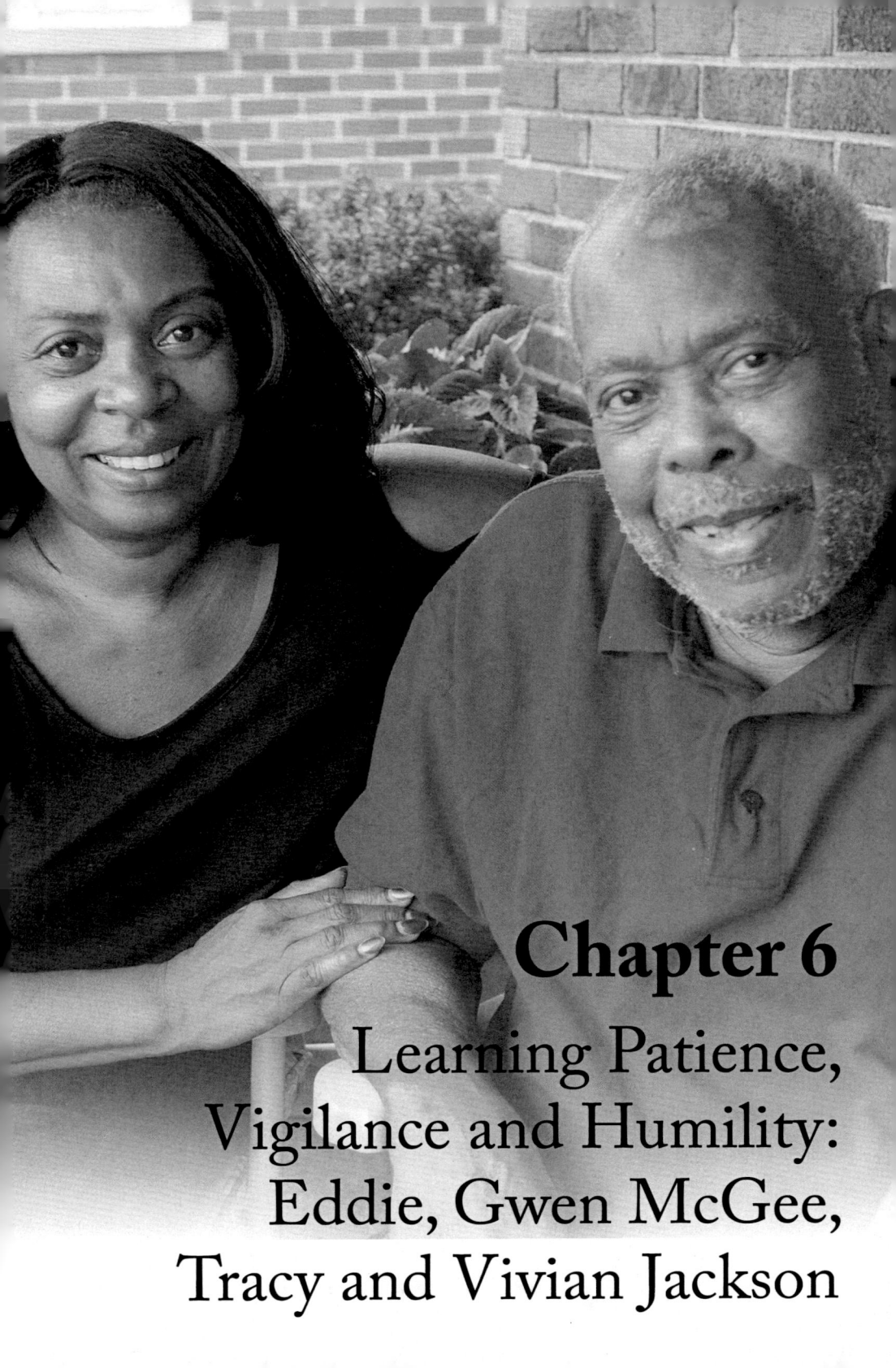

Chapter 6
Learning Patience, Vigilance and Humility: Eddie, Gwen McGee, Tracy and Vivian Jackson

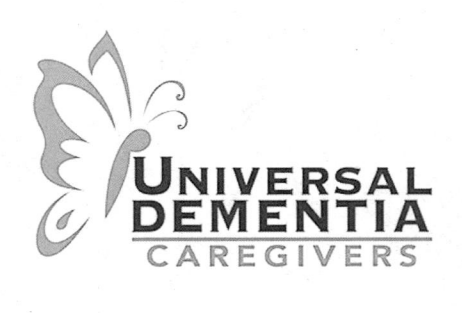

UNIVERSAL DEMENTIA
CAREGIVERS

www.universaldementia.org

Meet Eddie, Gwen McGee, Tracy and Vivian Jackson

Despite caring for two parents for nearly a decade, Gwen McGee never thought of herself as a caregiver. Then in 2018, when her mother had endured the many stages of dementia, Gwen started attending some support group meetings for people like her.

"How did I do all that?"

"I started understanding the role of a caregiver," says Gwen, 65. She realized her organizational skills and ability to identify resources from years working in foster care were especially valuable in her journey. So was her bachelor's degree in family life education and master's degree in families' studies, which gave her some acceptance during her mother's final days, she says. "I kind of knew what was going to happen."

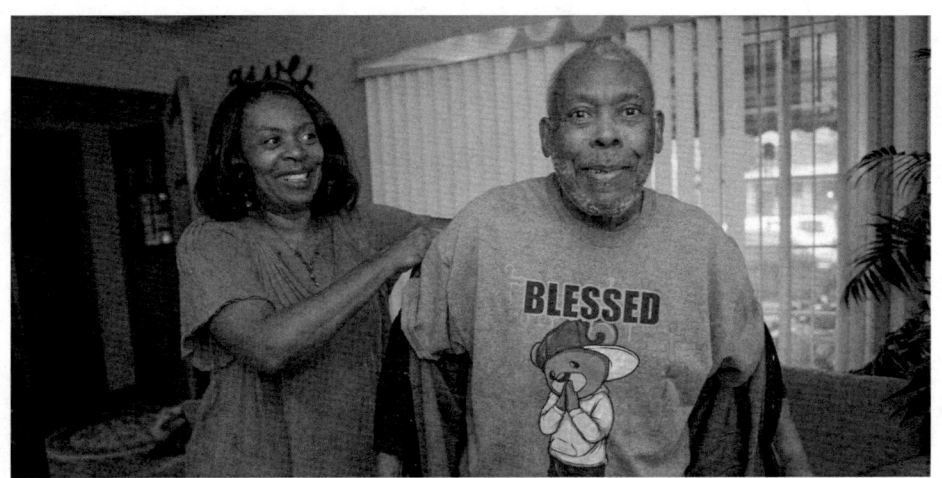

She thinks back now to something her mother's hospice nurse told her, "You made this easy." She didn't understand what that meant at

Chapter 6 - Learning Patience Vigilance and Humility -

the time. Her mother, Clara, had been bedridden for several months before her death at age 86 in April 2019. Clara required full-time care, everything from changing diapers and laundry to cooking, paying bills. "Today I think, how did I do all that?"

Gwen moved in with her parents in 2002 when she herself needed support. When it came to her mother's care, she never missed a beat. Gwen saw to every detail, from getting mom musical and physical therapy to identifying a chaplain and a massage therapist to meet her needs. That was the toughest time, says Gwen, whose father, Eddie, 90, recently received a dementia-related disorder diagnosis. "It was overwhelming," she expressed.

After A Spouse Dies

Now she hopes to do as well if not better for "Dad". He's known as "G Pop" or "Pop Pop" to his five grandchildren and nine great grandchildren. Dad clearly misses his wife of over 60 years. "Sometimes he asks where she is or says, 'I just saw her in the kitchen.' Other times he realizes she's gone.

His dementia worsened after her mother died and he suffered a series of seizures. Nonetheless, he still has some independence. He savors the big breakfasts Gwen makes for him and loves sitting on the front porch of their Detroit home admiring her garden. Last summer, he played ball with his great grandson in the backyard. He's a jack-of-all-trades who likes to stay busy. "I really just let him do his thing," Gwen says. Within reason, of course. "He often tries to use the lawnmower, and I have to talk him out of it."

Eddie, a former Marine who retired after 30 years at Chrysler, always had side jobs like finishing basements, she says. "I was his helper. I was a tomboy." Gwen grew up with three sisters (one has since passed away), and learned a lot from Eddie about how to fix things around the house. "Dad would always say: "Girl, you better come over here and let me teach you how to do that." It's been hard for him not to do those things anymore. Gwen recalls trying to hire someone to finish the basement and Dad said, "You and I could do it." They laughed about it together as she reminded him that remodeling was part of their past.

Shared Caregiving as a Family

While Gwen is the primary caregiver, she's had help from her siblings over the years. These days younger sister Tracy, who trains medical assistants, provides some of Dad's personal care

> When frustration mounts, Gwen relies on her own advice: "Let things go and know that it's not that person. Step back, go for a walk, go to another part of the house, and find ways to redirect the behavior."

like clipping his nails. Older sister, Vivian does what she can, often dropping off meals. Vivian also makes Gwen laugh. "She's awesome," Gwen explained, especially at encouraging her to take time off. Gwen, who misses traveling since the COVID-19 pandemic hit, gets her self-care by gardening, praying, and keeping a journal. And she keeps in

Chapter 6 - Learning Patience Vigilance and Humility - 53

mind a favorite slogan, "One day at a time."

Some days test Gwen more than others — usually when Eddie repeats things too many times or asks the same question over and over. It's also frustrating trying to get him to understand what is going on.

For example, on the morning of the interview for this book project, Dad woke up and pulled out his suit to dress for his grandson's wedding which was two weeks earlier.

"When I came back into the room he was dressed. I had to get on my phone and show him pictures that it had already happened. It usually doesn't turn into an argument but if I have something to do, my patience can get worn out."

Managing the Frustrations

When frustration mounts, Gwen relies on her own advice: "Let things go and know that it's not that person. Step back, go for a walk, go to another part of the house, and find ways to redirect the behavior." Perhaps more importantly, "Remember these are your parents. They cared for you from the very beginning. They always had your back no matter what."

Though scary, Dad's last time driving in 2018 did not result in any injury.

Dad was two hours late returning home from visiting Mom in a rehab center. He'd gotten lost once before. Gwen and her sisters immediately posted their concern to Facebook and were in the process of making a missing person's report when he walked in. "He said, he felt like he was in a dream and ended up downtown," recalls Gwen, who took his keys that night. He didn't argue.

If she has any regrets, it was a decision made during her mother's final days, three weeks before her death, when they couldn't wake her up. Rather than call hospice as instructed, they called an ambulance. "I think she would have gone peacefully," said Gwen. Instead, she returned home from the hospital with a large bed sore because they weren't turning her "like we do at home." Her mother couldn't verbalize or swallow and spent her last days filled with agitation, she says. "I don't want that for dad."

By this point, she's not too worried about Dad's care and his final days. She's also taken care of all the legal matters. "Everything is all good with the three girls and what he wants everybody to have." And then she somberly adds: "I've come to the acceptance, eventually, of what's going to happen."

It's one day at a time. "I do what I need to do daily. I make sure he's fed and take him to his daily appointments," she says. "I'm content." Even more, she says she feels blessed. "I consider this another Godly assignment."

DR. PAULA'S INSIGHTS:

1. **You must stay in the moment.** If you focus on the past, you feel bad and guilty. If you focus on the future, you worry about what's going to happen. Be present in the moment and focus on right now.

2. **Tap into Your Resources.** Learn the resources available for support as soon as possible. Chapter 12 in this book is full of useful information for caregivers.

3. **Self-Care is not Selfish.** You're doing a good job. Learn how to appreciate your importance to your loved one. Take good care of you and remember to only take it one day at a time.

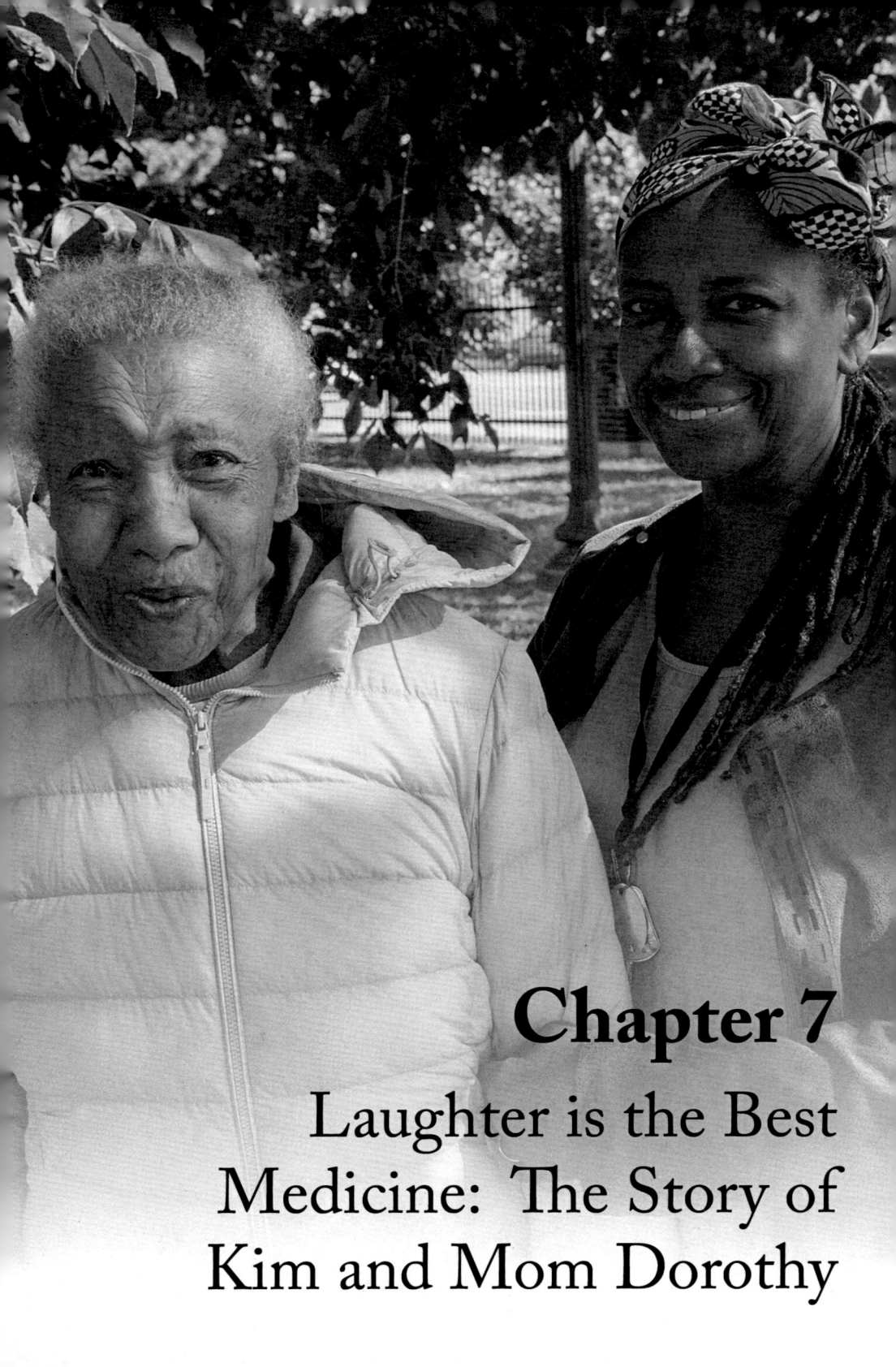

Chapter 7
Laughter is the Best Medicine: The Story of Kim and Mom Dorothy

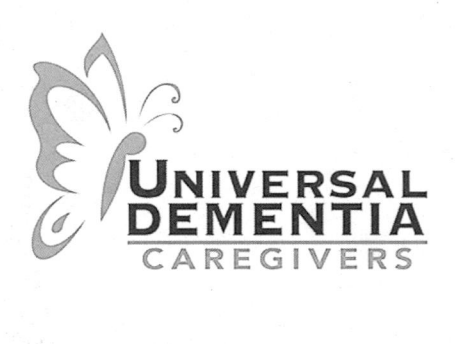

UNIVERSAL DEMENTIA CAREGIVERS

www.universaldementia.org

Meet Kim Ewing and Mom Dorothy

Kim Ewing does not think dementia is funny, but humor helps her cope.

While caregiving for her mother, Dorothy, who has Alzheimer's disease, they laugh heartily and often. "We actually wake up laughing because I do stupid things like open her door and it squeaks. She laughs first and we'll sit on the bed laughing."

It's a welcome change from earlier years when Kim was more likely to be crying or calling the Alzheimer's hotline saying she wished it would all be over. Now she sees the ridiculousness, mostly in herself, of asking her mother something she knows she can't answer because she has Alzheimer's. "Sometimes it feels like you're in a sitcom. Like the Alzheimer's parent and the child. That would be so hilarious."

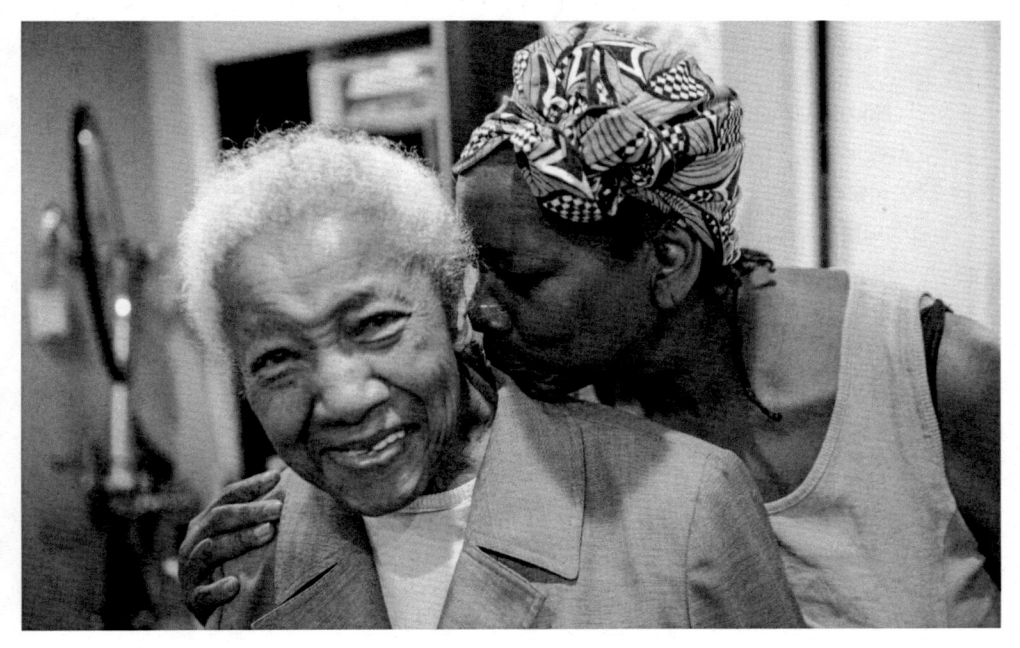

If laughter is good medicine, Kim, 64, can certainly use it. While devoting much of her life to caring for her family, she ignored her own health for too long.

Her care journey began with her grandmother, who also had Alzheimer's disease. She and Dorothy, now 85, cared for her together when Kim was in her 20s. Then around 2000, when her father was diagnosed with heart failure, life took another turn. Kim's father was an engineer who moved the family around the country for various jobs, including working on NASA's Apollo program. Kim, who was working as a record music industry publicist in New York City, left her job to help her mother care for her father in their Seattle home. Her mother was already showing early signs of Alzheimer's. There was never a doubt in Kim's mind that she'd care for her parents. "It was automatic," she says. "They gave me my life."

> If she has any advice for other caregivers, she would say to learn everything you can about the disease and get ready to give up a lot of you. But, she assures, you will not be lost, "You will find you and you will find you – stronger."

Family was always important to Kim, the oldest of three siblings. Her two younger brothers predeceased her father. Losing their sons took a huge toll, says Kim. "That kind of contributed to my parents going down after that."

After her father died in 2010, Kim says she kind of forgot about her mother's dementia as she saw how focused Dorothy was on her husband's care. "I thought she was fine." Then one day, frustrated with so many details of moving out of their house, Kim tried to get her mother to focus. "I said, 'what's going on? You need to help me here.'" Dorothy replied, "You never let me do anything! All I want to do is just go outside!"

That's when it hit Kim. "It started right there," she says. She decided to settle in Detroit, where Kim was born. "I just kept hearing voices like, 'y'all need to go back home,' 'take her home.' So, I said, 'Okay, we're going home.'" Home was back to Detroit.

Today they're like roommates with lots of family photos spread throughout their colorful apartment. Seeing her family's faces around her helps, says Kim, who feels encouraged spiritually. "My father and brothers are ever present in my spirit providing guidance."

While Kim gets some support from her cousins, she mostly relies on a health aide named Jessica who's been with them for more than a year now. "She feels like a daughter to me," says Kim, who never had children and calls Jessica her caregiver, daughter, and granddaughter to her mother. "Her kids love my mother. It's just like having a family."

"I'm adopted into this family," says Jessica. Kim jokes that her mother likes Jessica better."

Dorothy, who sits in a chair, her gray hair in a tidy bun, smiles sweetly as Kim chats but doesn't speak much the past few years. A working woman who raised three kids, Dorothy "took care of everything," recalls Kim. Now she takes care to ensure Dorothy eats healthy and stays active with walks around the block. "I plan for her to not be in a wheelchair or a walker because she is always active," she says. "Dorothy is much like a child now, I often feel like her mother."

Kim was unsure how to handle that role at first. She recalls her mother behaving in ways that if she did it as a child, Dorothy would grab her arm. Kim wondered, "Should I do that?" Now she's more comfortable in her position. "I tell her when to go to bed. If she wants to stay up I let her," says Kim, who's discovered some gifts during this time. "I've never been a mother but sometimes I look at her and I can tell what the feeling is like. Like, oh my God, I just love you. And I can see how a parent would do anything for that baby."

In fact, since Dorothy stopped speaking, it's opened space for a "spiritual soulful connection... A kind of knowing when she needs to go to the bathroom, when she needs a hug, when she needs me to sit in the room with her while watching TV. It's not just being with her but everything else you deal with. That's been a really strong gift given to me."

Kim's main challenge now is caring for herself. "I've neglected myself a lot, for a long time. Especially when taking care of mom and dad." For years she was out of shape, not eating right, not sleeping. "I was a functioning wreck," she says. Once she started getting healthy — working out, losing weight, seeing the doctor — she discovered some health issues she's now watching. It was a wakeup call. "Maybe all this built up when I was taking care of them," she says. "I thought I was like Superwoman."

One of her greatest acts of self-care now is gardening in their apartment building's courtyard. It's a love her grandmother instilled in her as a child, she says, "digging in the dirt."

If she has any advice for other caregivers, she would say to learn everything you can about the disease and get ready to give up a lot of you. But, she assures, you will not be lost, "You will find you and you will find you – stronger."

DR. PAULA'S INSIGHTS:

After reading **Kim Ewing's** story, I want you to note the following key takeaways:

1. **Humor is a game changer.** There are some common strategies that caregivers use as a means of coping. In Kim's situation, she uses humor and it helps her keep from crying. You must find ways to cope to be successful as a caregiver. Reading, exercising, praying, challenging your thoughts, socializing, meditating are all strategies for consideration. One important thing is accepting the role of caregiver. You must accept the responsibilities and prepare yourself for the challenges and the joys ahead.

2. **Caregivers have more talent and skills than they ever realized.** They often take their talents for granted. Kim is an exceptional artist. Her gifts show in how she decorates the home, prepares Mom's food in a holistic way and keeps the garden. She ensures that Mom is honored and has become an outstanding advocate for getting Mom's needs met.

3. **You can not do it alone.** Kim was honest about her journey -- "I was a functioning wreck. I was trying to be a superwoman. You cannot do it alone." Allowing others to assist is difficult for many caregivers. Some believe that no one can care for their loved one as well as themselves. I tell caregivers this is probably true, but you will burnout trying to do everything yourself. Simply ensure that others who assist create a space of honor and safety. Learning how to cope and understanding the importance of seeking help is vital.

Chapter 8

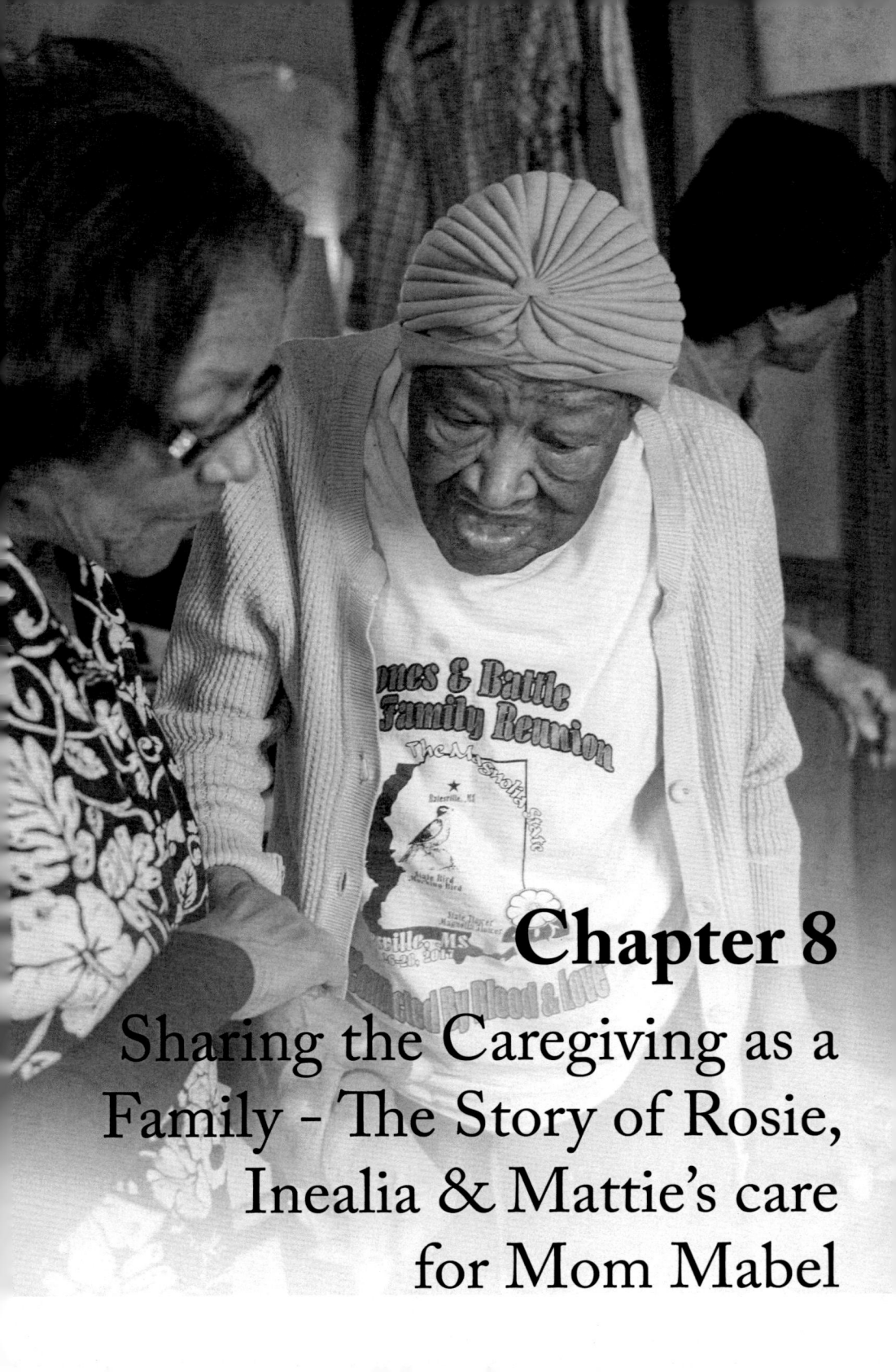

Sharing the Caregiving as a Family - The Story of Rosie, Inealia & Mattie's care for Mom Mabel

www.universaldementia.org

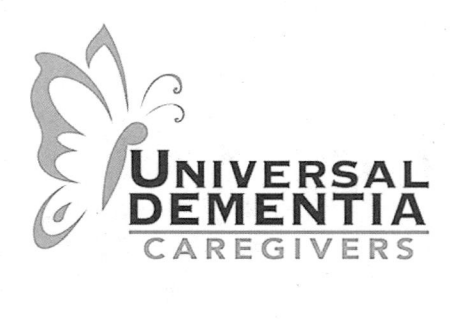

Meet Rosie, Inealia, Mattie and Mom Mabel

A combination of happenstance and loving commitment found three sisters – Rosie Lee, Inealia, and Mattie Pearl -- in their 70s, once again, living under their mother's roof.

Together the siblings care for 96-year-old Mom Mabel Lee Benson, who suffers from dementia. One by one they moved into Mom Mabel's Detroit home of nearly 60 years, never once considering putting her in a nursing home, which was an added blessing during the Covid-19 pandemic.

For the three sisters, there was never any hesitation. It was just a part of their duty to take care of their parents and loved ones. Rosie Lee Jones, 77, a retired aide who provided patient

> This time together has given the sisters a chance to reflect both on their mother and themselves.

support for over 30 years at Harper Hospital in Detroit, has cared for Mom Mabel the longest, about five years longer than her siblings. She handles most of her mother's personal care like bathing and dressing, while her sisters focus on other tasks.

Inealia Potts, 74, a soft-spoken former second-grade school teacher, moved in after separating from her husband in 2017. The baby of the family, Mattie Pearl Hunter, 72, a longtime executive secretary who likes to joke and lives with limitations from a stroke years ago, moved in after her husband of nearly 50 years died in 2020. Her sons didn't want her to be alone. Together the two do most of the cooking, cleaning, laundry, and shopping.

Of course, the sisters — all mothers themselves blessing Mom Mabel with 12 grandchildren between them — have had to adapt to living together for the first time since they were kids. While they show few signs of conflict as they surround their mother in her cozy living room, they admit they have their disagreements. But there's no time for grudges. They always make up within the hour, they say. Plus, getting along is just part of their faith. "We're all Christians. We know how the Lord would have us conduct ourselves," says Inealia.

Keeping the peace is also something they do for their mother as well as for their own sakes, says Rosie Lee, "You make her life better, you make your life better." There is a clear reverence each has for Mom Mabel, who was born in rural Mississippi and never had more than a fourth-grade education. She married their dad and had the girls down south, where they worked and picked cotton until the family moved to Detroit in 1957.

"She was tough," says Mattie. "My dad brought his check home, and he got an allowance. She took care of all the bills. My dad had excellent credit because of her." Mom Mabel was a hard worker, too, mostly as a homemaker especially on Sundays when she laid out an elaborate meal for the family. She also enjoyed tending to her big backyard garden. Once the girls were teenagers, she took jobs cleaning the church once a week and cleaned homes for various clients. Mom Mabel was not one to sit idle.

Indeed, admitted Mattie, "We used to tease her that she'd break things to fix them." They laugh but there is some sadness there, too. Mom Mabel will often express a desire to wash dishes, which her daughters agree she can not do because she has difficulty standing. She told her daughters, "I worked all my life." Yet, they don't have any work for her.

This journey has had its challenges, especially as Mom Mabel's health declines.

Rosie Lee has noticed how things have changed. "I'm more responsible than I used to be. Mom used to take care of practically everything. She used to fix me something to eat. Now I have to fix something for us both and put out her clothes."

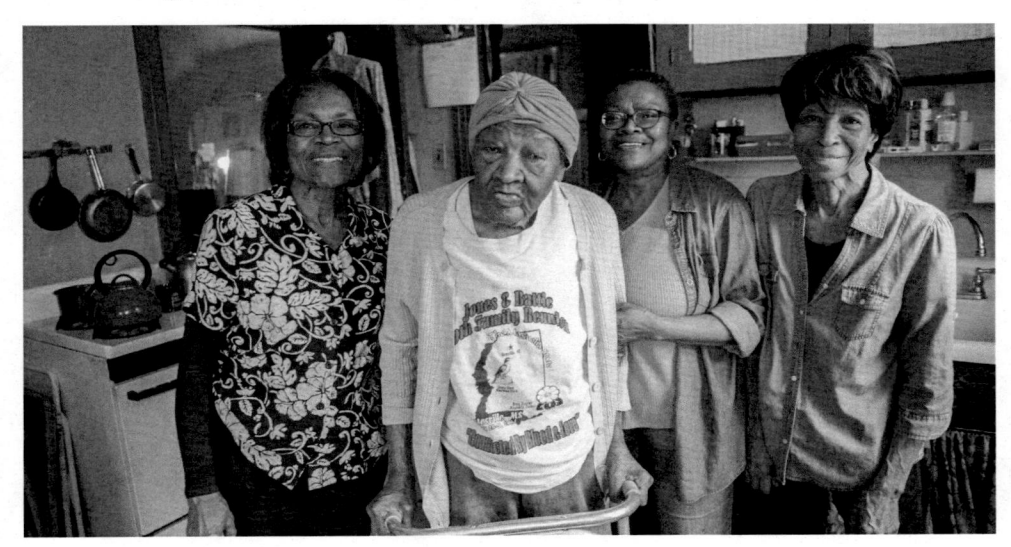

Rosie Lee admits it's hard to see her mother as she is today: weaker than usual, dozing off in her wheelchair with her head down to her knees. "But I don't show it. I talk regular, like, 'You want some breakfast?'"

This time together has given the sisters a chance to reflect both on their mother and themselves. Inealia contemplates aloud the Universal Dementia motto shared with all caregivers during bootcamps, "To honor who they are and to love who they are and to welcome who they become is how I best cope." She then looks to her mother, seated beside her. "She was a good mother," she says, as she shares a memory of when she got her first job in high school. "I had to be at work at 6 am and she would dress up as a man and walk me to the bus stop." Inealia is still amazed. "She did that. She's done so much. She never ever refused to watch my children if I had something to do. There's nothing for us to do but assist her now."

When asked what advice they can offer to others in their shoes, the sisters agree, simply, "Love is the first ingredient."

It's clear they also recognize the value of self-care as they share concern for Rosie Lee. "She has a tendency not to take care of herself," says Mattie. It's something a visiting high school friend of Rosie Lee's echoes from the next room. "I want her to get out. But she loves her mama," he says. "It's hard to get her to step away."

If Rosie Lee dotes too much on Mom Mabel, sometimes doing things she could do for herself, she admits it's partly out of guilt as the one daughter who caused a bit of concern for her parents growing up. "I wasn't bad-bad," she explains. "But I'm trying to make up for some of that."

Mostly the sisters want to honor this time with Mom Mabel, a woman they recall as so talkative and even a bit of a comedian. "I make jokes as we set the table and I say foolish stuff. And she laughs," says Mattie. Rosie Lee cherishes the times her mother recognizes her, saying: "Rosie, stop that," or "Rosie, don't do this," she says. "I can tell she still loves us."

As for Inealia, her mother's presence is enough: "I just enjoy sitting with her and talking to her. Spending quiet time together."

DR. PAULA'S INSIGHTS:

After reading **Mom Mabel's** story, I want you to note the following key takeaways:

1. **You must see the beauty of your loved one at every stage of the dementia journey, and lay aside your personal agenda.** Mom Mabel is blessed to have her three daughters prioritizing her care and living together in peace under one roof.

2. **Caregiving is a natural progression of life.** Many families often see the role of caregiver as a duty and obligation. In Mom Mabel's case, her daughters view it as a privilege to walk the last journey with their mom.

3. **Focus on what matters most for your loved one.** Many families struggle with who's in charge, who has the power, and who makes the decisions. But at the end of the day, all decisions must be rooted in what is best for your loved one and their needs.

Chapter 9
One Day at a Time - The Story of Doris "Dot"

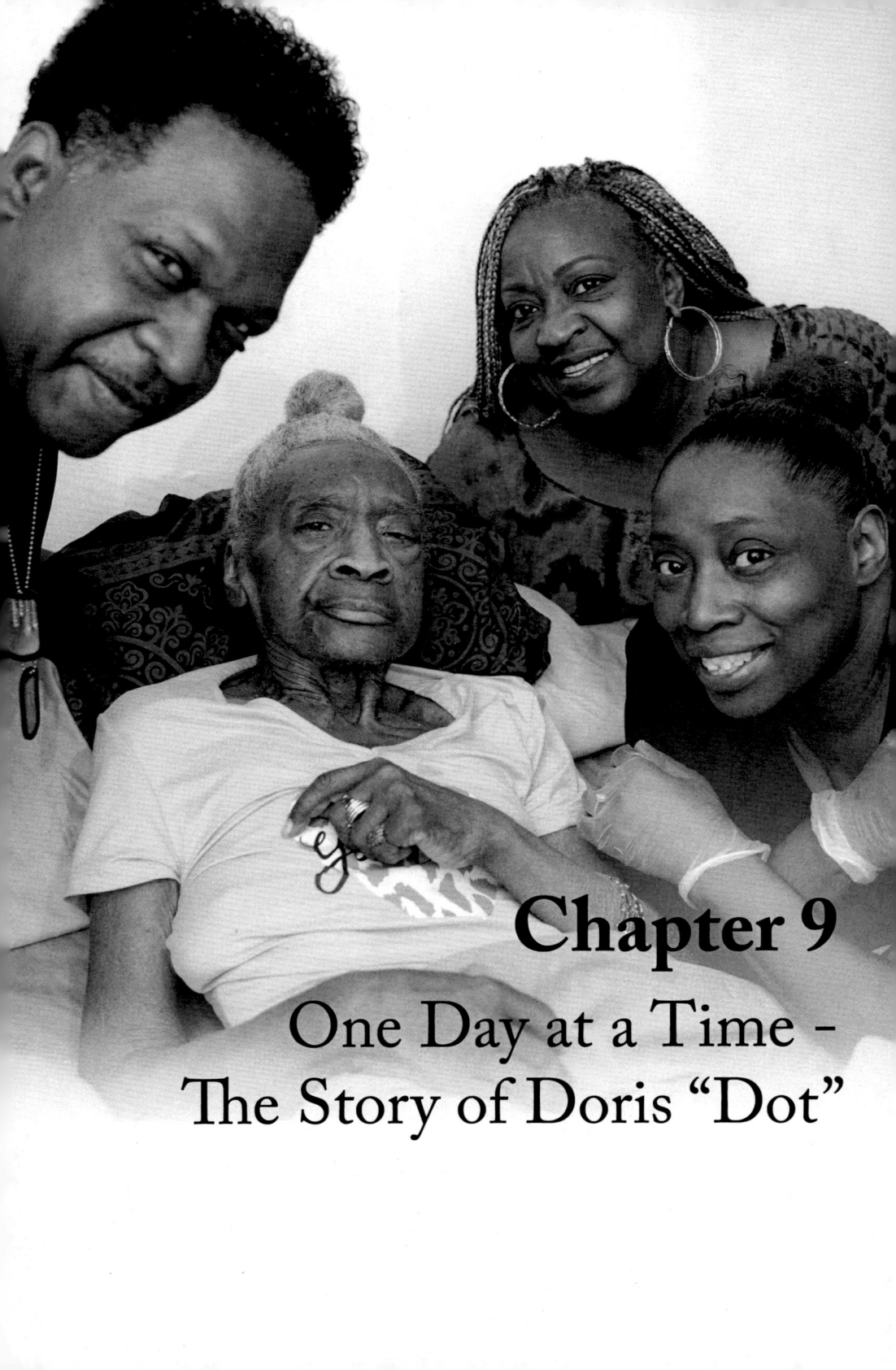

UNIVERSAL
DEMENTIA
CAREGIVERS

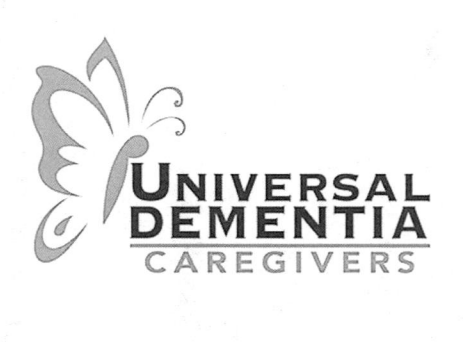

www.universaldementia.org

Meet Doris "Dot" Stanley

Years before Doris "Dot" Stanley was diagnosed with dementia, she was a beautician. She favored fancy clothes and was particularly well-mannered and no-nonsense.

"She was the auntie who didn't play," says her niece and caregiver Tia Wortheen with a laugh. Doris, or "my T" as she calls her, was the first person she ever saw eat pizza with a fork and a knife. "I was like a tomboy. She used to say, 'You need to start wearing dresses.' I won that battle."

Doris' sister and caregiver, Deborah Hayes, says "Dot," 79, the eldest of six siblings, was that sister she looked up to. "She was always beautiful and had everything going for her. She taught me about designer clothes and where to shop." Today, Deborah, 64, is mindful of that person when handling her finances or picking out colorful tops for her to wear. "I think, 'No, she wouldn't wear that,'" she says. "Like, what would she want?"

For Tia, it's enough just being there for her aunt. "I'm doing what I'm supposed to do. That makes me the happiest." Adding that she can't imagine putting anyone in a facility especially during the COVID-19 pandemic. "To see them through a window or not be able to talk to them? That wouldn't work for me."

The two women never questioned that Doris would be anywhere but in her own home. "We always knew we'd care for one another," says

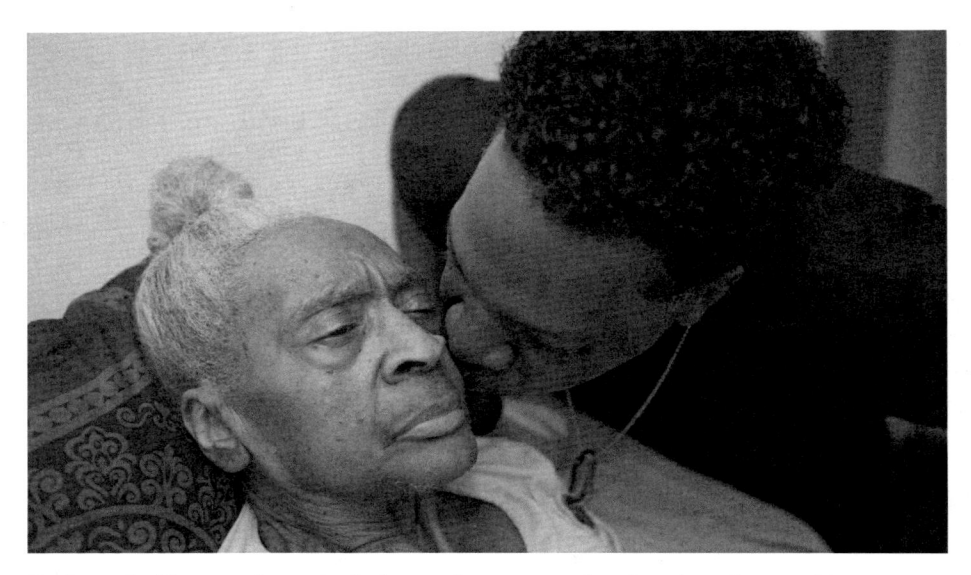

Deborah. "It was handed down because that's what I saw. My mom cared for everyone." The women know the sacrifices. Deborah, who lives nearby, retired in January 2020 as a mortgage loan analyst to be more available to care for her mother, who died in December – that same year in the same home in Detroit.

Tia, meanwhile, has been caring for her mother, Jean, 75 (Deborah and Doris's sister) since 2001. She left a factory job in 2012 to be available full-time and now lives with Jean on the second floor of the "family home" while Doris and her son, Reginald "Reggie," 59, live on the main floor.

But even with family all around, they didn't recognize when Doris showed early signs of dementia. At the time, Deborah's mother was helping Doris by taking care of the bills and making sure she was eating.

But as Doris's condition worsened, she became combative and stopped taking her medicine. "We saw the toll it was taking on mom," says Deborah. "You could tell she was getting tired." Then one day the house smelled of gas. Doris was trying to cook. "We had to take the knobs off the stove. And it kind of hit me, this is serious."

Then the family started researching and learning about dementia. "Even Reggie finally got it," says Deborah of her nephew who was slow to accept how severe Dot's condition truly was for her safety. Now he's part of her care team. These days Dot, who no longer speaks and spends her days in bed in a room with a TV running 24/7, gets round-the-clock care from her loved ones.

> Now healthcare providers come into their home and have trained the caregivers to do things like treat bed sores. "We are learning every day," says Deborah.

Deborah says she is more like an assistant to Tia in the day-to-day tasks, usually arriving in the morning to help with bathing and cleaning. Reggie likes to cook. They have it down; a solid routine. So much so Deborah says they barely know what to do with sister Cynthia, one of the four surviving siblings. She calls all the time to offer support: 'I'm here if you need me.'

Tia does more of the heavy-lifting but is also gentle, says Deborah, the heavier-handed one. "I'm like: Let's get it over with," she laughs. She's also "the one out on the street," whether finding something

Doris will eat or their favorite brand of pull-ups. Besides cooking, Reggie is very attentive to "abnormal body things," says Deborah. "He'll take a picture and say, 'Have you seen this?'" Tia laughs: "He notices everything."

They have a rhythm now, but they had their challenges in the beginning. It was hard at first to accept Doris as bedridden; her legs now maintained in a folded position. The women kept trying to move her, get her to the bathroom, get her to sit in a chair, get her on her feet. "We were making her walk. We'd say, 'You can do it.' We even pushed her in a chair through the house," says Deborah. At some point it hit us, "why are we putting her through this?"

Around that time, late 2020, they saw Doris was having some pain. They took her to urgent care and learned she had a fracture. Then that December, Doris was having Parkinson's-like symptoms, so they called for a video conference with her doctor. When he was not available, the doctor who took their call happened to ask what they knew about palliative care, which prioritizes comfort over cures. Deborah immediately thought it meant "hospice was right around the corner. She soon learned that it was just to make her comfortable and "not to read anything more into it." Now healthcare providers come into their home and have trained the caregivers to do things like treat bed sores. "We are learning every day," says Deborah. "We even got a pillow to put between her legs. You're constantly thinking, what could make her comfortable?"

Though Doris no longer speaks, she communicates. "Doris eats good for Tia. She eats for me, but not as good," says Deborah. "She won't eat for Cynthia."

Nothing beats Doris seeing her grandchildren, says Tia. "She really lights up."

As for their own self-care, Deborah looks out for Tia. "I get to go out and sleep in my own bed, so I ask, 'Do you want to go to the park? See your boyfriend?' He comes to the house for date night. Tia laughs about it but admits it's hard to take a break. "I'm very territorial."

When asked to offer advice, Dot's care team stressed having patience and being vigilant. "You have to learn their moves, know when they're not feeling well." In Tia's eyes, a caregiver must have heart. "If you don't care it's not going to work."

Humility is important, too, says Deborah. "Some mornings it's raining, and I'd love to just stay at home. And you can't. It's not about you anymore."

DR. PAULA'S INSIGHTS:

After reading Doris "Dot" Stanley's story, I want you to note the following key takeaways:

1. **Honor who they were.** When caregiving for a loved one with dementia you must know them to honor their needs. Dot's family took great care to consider her personality and preferences as they served her.

2. **Be a great detective.** Listen for the unspoken. See past the behavior. Your loved one has unmet needs such as desiring independence and engagement just like you. They just no longer have the ability to communicate this in words.

3. **Family does not have to be blood.** Friends, neighbors, church members and more can all add to the care of your loved one. It's important to have others to help address the feeling of isolation.

Chapter 10

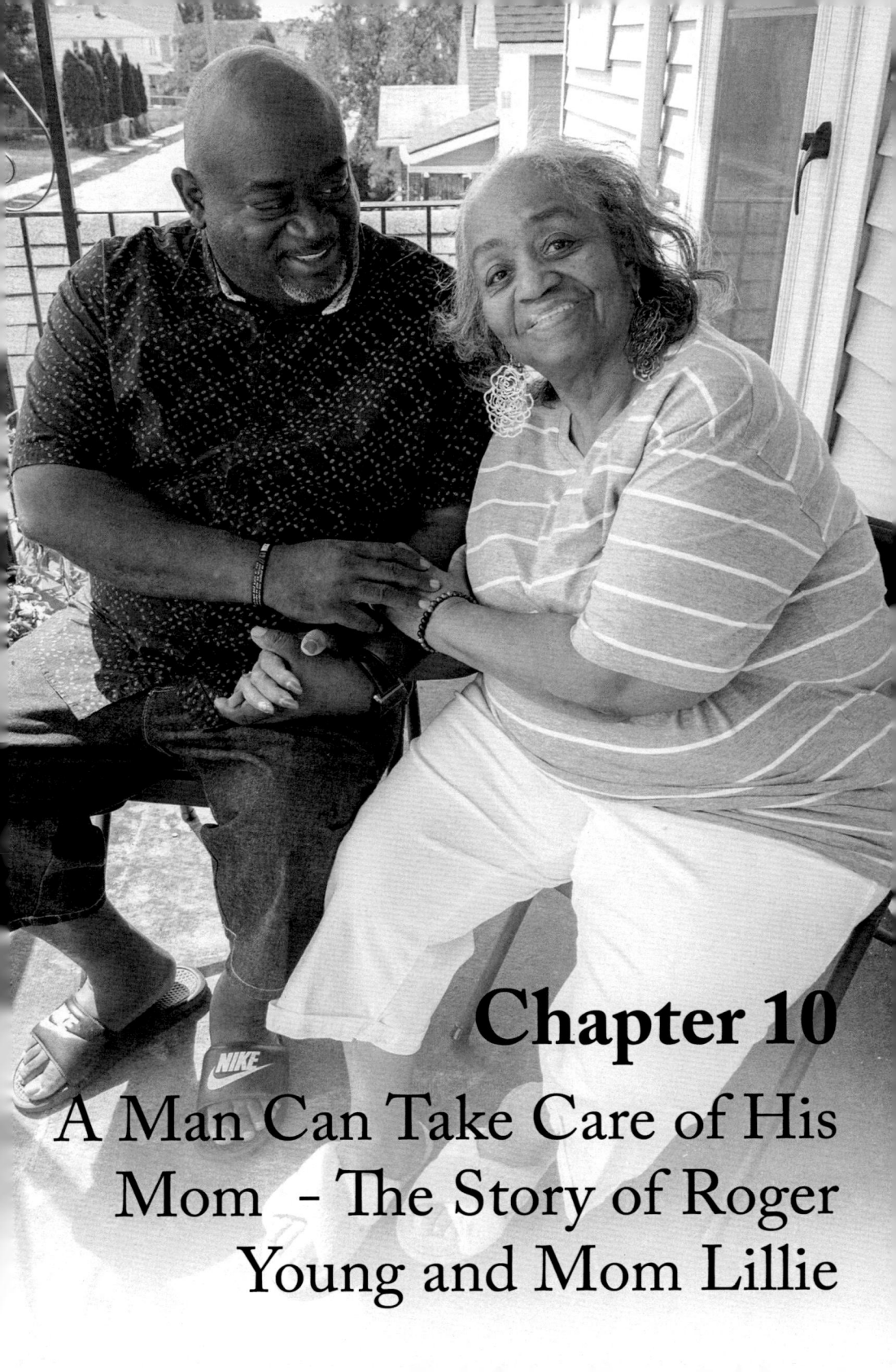

A Man Can Take Care of His Mom - The Story of Roger Young and Mom Lillie

UNIVERSAL
DEMENTIA
CAREGIVERS

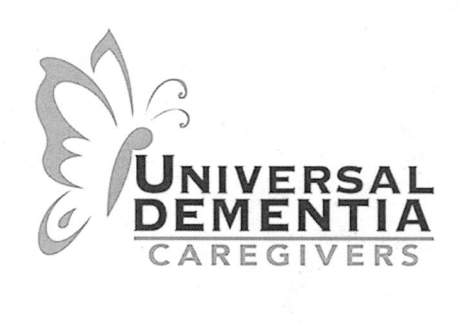

www.universaldementia.org

Meet Roger Young and Mom Lillie

Roger Young's mother, Lillie, taught him well.

Growing up in Hamtramck he saw how she took care of everyone, not just her three children and two step-kids but "half the kids in Detroit." And, despite being one of 10 siblings, Lillie was the one who cared for both of her parents in their final years. "We never really had our mother to ourselves," he says.

It's just what you did.

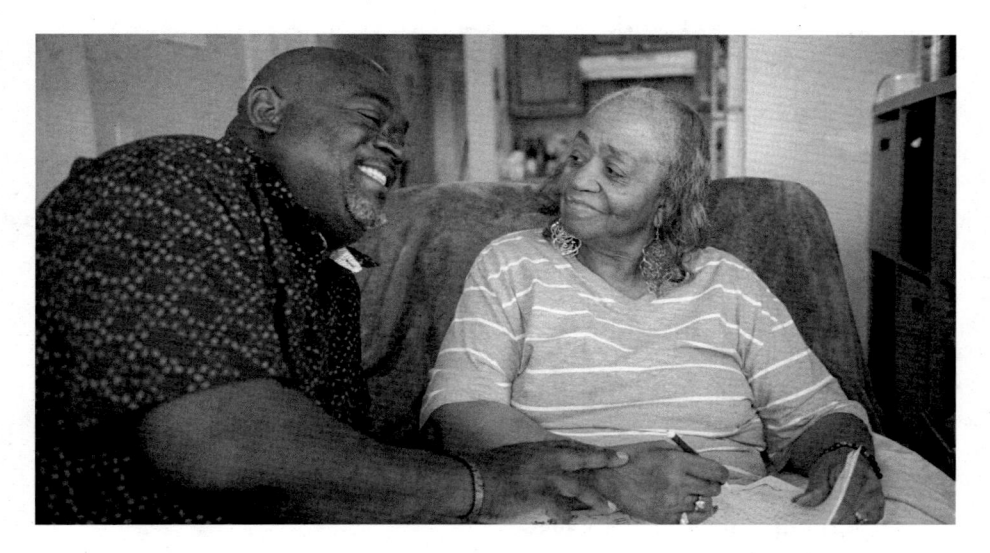

A Family Legacy of Care

"She instilled that in me," says Roger, now 62, the oldest child raised by the single mother. He cared for his siblings over the years, cousins, too, as well as aunts, nieces, nephews and even the neighborhood kids, keeping them off the street.

So when his mother, Lillie, now 83, needed help, he was there.

"I've always been super close to my mom," says Roger, who never had children of his own. "I'm used to taking care of people."

It was hard at first to face when Lillie was diagnosed with dementia and Alzheimer's Disease.

She was "the rock" of the family, "the matriarch" who worked as an X-ray technician and was treasurer for her church. Always handling things, he says. "I never thought she'd get to a place where she couldn't handle her stuff."

Facing the Caregiving Requirements

It started about 10 years ago.

Although Roger saw Lillie daily — both lived in Hamtramck — nothing was obvious right away. Nor was it for his two siblings who were living with her during some of those years.

It didn't help that Lillie was always private. "I never knew what was going on with her," Roger says.

But then he began noticing things. She wasn't paying some bills while double paying others. She was also driving erratically, one day stopping in the middle of Eight Mile Road for no apparent reason. And then people were coming to the house to collect on bills. "I thought, 'What is going on?'"

By the time Lillie's house went into foreclosure, she was living alone. Roger tried unsuccessfully to get it back. In 2015, he moved her in with him. "We'll figure something out," he told her.

Roger cried for two years before he started to learn about her disease and how he could best support her.

Today, with an aide to help with bathing and other tasks, Roger does pretty much everything for Lillie, from cooking to driving, to cleaning and brushing her shoulder length gray hair.

Lillie doubted him at first. She would always say, "You don't know anything about being a woman." Roger laughs as Lillie, sitting beside him at the kitchen table, gently swats him. "He learned," she says.

Making the Time Worthwhile

Besides taking care of his mother, Roger has completed a certification in aging mastery while running a catering business. Lillie helps.

> Sometimes I get her up to dance with me. So whatever struggles I have it seems worth it to have that time with her.

"She does all my cutting and prepping. She enjoys doing it and I appreciate it because it's a lot of work." She also folds clothes after he does the wash.

If anything is typical about their daily lives, Roger says it's when she sits in her chair with the purple throw and does her puzzles while he sits across from her and maybe listens to some jazz.

Lillie loves word puzzles. "I want to keep my mind going," she says. "I know it's gone down, but if I do puzzles and reading, it won't go down much faster."

Music is something the two can share. Sometimes after dinner they have music nights, says Roger. "Music amazes her. I do YouTube, '50s and '60s music, from her era, and we listen for hours. She loves jazz, too, and I play all her favorites. Sometimes I get her up to dance with me. So whatever struggles I have it seems worth it to have that time with her."

Facing Frustrations Head On

Roger knows what to do and how to advise others new to caregiving for someone with dementia.

One lesson he's learned: "They don't know what they're doing or where they're at mentally because that part of their brain is no longer there. I cannot make her see or do something that is not there. Once you understand that, you can put it in action," he says. "Step back, exhale, take a five minute break and then start over. Otherwise you react out of frustration."

Roger recently reacted in frustration, he says, "going off in a way I never went off on my mom before." He was hollering and hitting the table with his hand so hard it hurt the next day. "And then I walked away. I should have walked away first. And who knows what she thinks."

He says one thing that frustrates him lately is that Lillie hides food she doesn't want to eat in a napkin during meals. He says it drives him crazy because she knows it's wrong because she's sneaking it. "I would rather she just say she won't eat it."

Then he takes a moment to reflect on his emotions. "Everyone has the fear that their loved one will forget them. Mine is that she will stop eating," he says, concerned that all she eats lately is cookies and juice. "I'm afraid she'll stop eating like her mom and dad."

The Power of Touch

Roger, who's had his own recent health issues and cut back on volunteering at his church, knows self-care is important. He reaches for Lillie's left hand to show how the power of touch can soothe them both.

"When I touch her like this it's such a soft, sentimental moment," he says, gently stroking her hand with his thumb. "I don't know what she's getting out of it but I feel just as calm. It's a powerful tool."

Meanwhile, he tries to accept what is, which is always changing. Lillie doesn't want to go out as much these days, but he keeps making the effort. "Sometimes I take her out and we ride and drive." He'll take her to Belle Isle and show her how Detroit has changed. "We go to lunch and have a nice time," he says. "I try to make sure she can still do life."

DR. PAULA'S INSIGHTS:

After reading Roger Young and his mother Lillie's story, I want you to note the following key takeaways:

1. **Feeling paralyzed in the pain is not uncommon.** Roger shared he cried for two years before he sought help, educated himself, took classes and joined a support group to better care for his mother. He also sought respite care for himself. This is such a good example of self care.

2. **They remember how you made them feel.** Roger's mom forgot his name at times. He stayed connected with her through regular touch and massage activities. When your loved ones words no longer make sense, you can connect with their heart and spirit. The best action at times is to simply be present.

3. **Love and commitment are more important than your skills.** Roger learned a son can care for his mother. He partnered in the care of his mother with her on the caregiving journey. It's not about the gender, but about the love of one human being towards another.

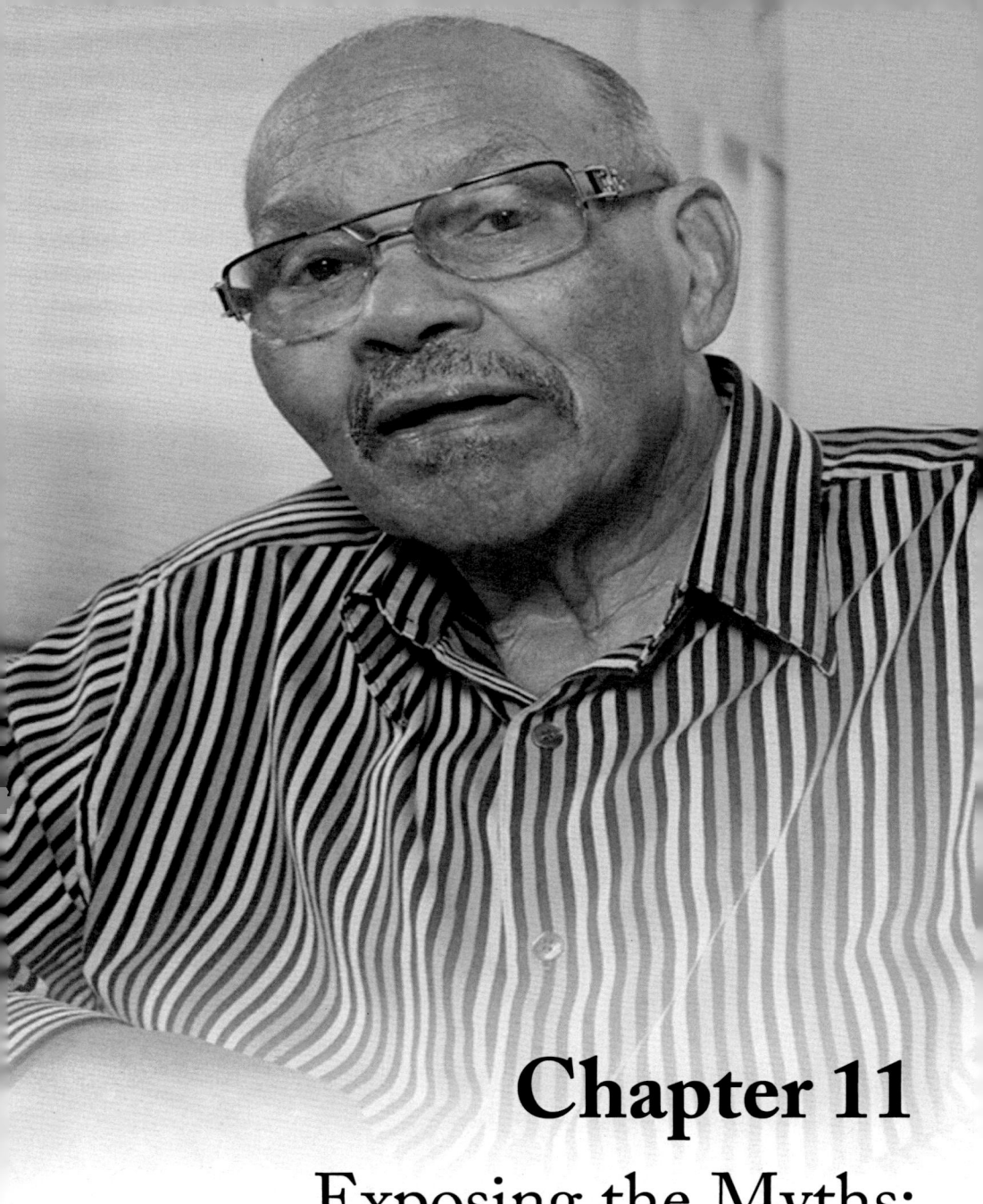

Chapter 11
Exposing the Myths: Understanding Alzheimer's and Dementia

www.universaldementia.org

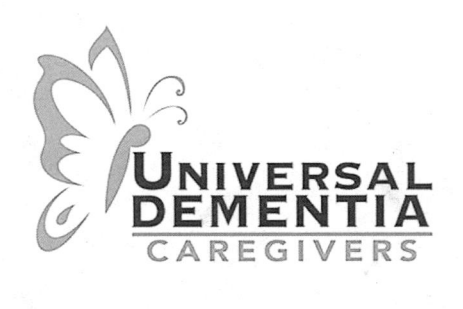

Now that you've laughed, cried and related to eight Detroit families coping with a loved one living with dementia, let's dive into demystifying common thoughts about dementia and Alzheimer's disease by first taking this quick quiz.

Myth Or Fact - Take the Quiz
(See page 100 for the correct answers)
1. Memory loss is a normal part of aging.
2. Dementia and Alzheimer's are the same thing.
3. Dementia only affects older people.
4. Dementia is a mental illness.
5. The cases of Alzheimer's are higher in communities of color.
6. Memory loss is a sign of Alzheimer's.
7. Alzheimer's can be prevented.
8. Taking supplements can prevent dementia. Vitamins and memory boosters can prevent Alzheimer's disease.
9. You should correct a person living with dementia when they make a verbal mistake.
10. It's not unusual for loved one with dementia to make false accusations against you.
11. There are some things that mimic dementia.
12. Flu shots increase the risk of dementia.
13. Treatments are available to stop the progression of Alzheimer's.
14. Visiting a person with dementia is not worth it because they quickly forget you were there.
15. Individuals affected by dementia cannot communicate what they want.
16. All people who have Alzheimer's disease become violent and aggressive.
17. Caregivers are the second invisible patient.
18. Some key issues need to be addressed asap to ensure loved one(s) are cared for properly.

Getting to the truth and exposing the myths

How many times have you heard someone joke about having 'old-timers' disease when they momentarily forget something? Dementia is a general term for decline in mental functioning that is severe enough to interfere with your daily activities. It impacts memory, language, reasoning, judgment, etc. Alzheimer's is a specific type of dementia disease and much more than temporarily forgetting where you placed your keys or glasses. Alzheimer's is the most common dementia disease accounting for 60-80% of dementia diseases.

Breaking Down Dementia

Dementia is an umbrella term for loss of memory and other abilities. Dementia is not a single disease; it's an overall term describing a group of symptoms — that can cover a wide range of conditions, including Alzheimer's disease. Alzheimer's is the most common cause of dementia related disease. Learning about dementia, its progression and symptoms can empower you to live with Alzheimer's or help a loved one who is coping with the disease.

Many different types of dementia diseases exist. That is why it is so important to obtain a diagnosis from a neurologist. A number of conditions mimic dementia. So I encourage you to avoid labeling yourself or a loved one. Instead, rely upon and seek professional assistance as soon as possible.

Alzheimer's is Not a Normal Part of Aging

In 1906, German physician Dr. Alois Alzheimer first described "a peculiar disease" — one of profound memory loss and microscopic brain changes — a disease we now know as Alzheimer's.

Alzheimer's is not a normal part of aging. Many people believe that the disease is just about memory loss, but it involves so much more. Alzheimer's worsens over time. It's a progressive disease, where dementia symptoms gradually worsen over several years. In its early stages, memory loss is mild, but with late-stage Alzheimer's, individuals can lose the ability to carry on a conversation and respond to their environment.

As Alzheimer's advances through the brain it leads to increasingly severe symptoms, including disorientation, mood and behavior changes; deepening confusion about events, time and place; suspicions about family, friends and professional caregivers; more serious memory loss and behavior changes; and difficulty speaking, walking and swallowing.

Symptoms of Alzheimer's

Alzheimer's is a complex disease and scientists don't know yet what causes it. The most common early symptom of Alzheimer's is difficulty remembering or short-term memory loss.

Just like the rest of our bodies, our brains change as we age. Most of us notice some slowed thinking and occasional problems with remembering certain things. However, serious memory loss, confusion and other major changes in the way our minds work may be a sign that brain cells are failing.

People with memory loss or other possible signs of Alzheimer's may find it hard to recognize they have a problem. Signs of dementia may be more obvious to family members or friends. Surprisingly, people who visit their doctor complaining of memory loss might actually be depressed, not dementia. Earlier diagnosis and intervention methods are improving dramatically, and treatment options and sources of support can improve quality of life.

On average, a person with Alzheimer's lives 4 to 8 years after diagnosis but can live 20 years, depending on the person. Each person is different and requires 'person centered care.' After a nearly 20-year dry spell in new treatments for Alzheimer's disease, the Food and Drug Administration (FDA) just approved a new Alzheimer's medication, Aduhelm (aducanumab). This very expensive treatment drug is developed by Biogen, with an expected annual price tag of $56,000. While the scientific community debates the evidence of the effectiveness of this new drug, there is great concern that particularly Medicare patients will never be able to even try it because the pricing is so cost prohibitive.

Alzheimer's and The Brain

Microscopic changes in the brain begin long before the first signs of memory loss.

The brain has 100 billion nerve cells (neurons). Each nerve cell connects with many others to form communication networks. Groups of nerve cells have special jobs. Some are involved in thinking, learning and remembering. Others help us see, hear and smell.

To do their work, brain cells operate like tiny factories. They receive supplies, generate energy, construct equipment and get rid of waste. Cells also process and store information and communicate with other cells. Keeping everything running requires coordination as well as large amounts of fuel and oxygen. The brain is a magnificent, complicated and wondrous thing.

Scientists believe Alzheimer's disease prevents parts of a cell's factory from running well. They are not sure where the trouble starts. But just like a real factory, backups and breakdowns in one system cause problems in other areas. As damage spreads, cells lose their ability to do their jobs and eventually die, causing irreversible changes in the brain.

Alzheimer's currently has no cure. There is a worldwide effort underway to find better ways to treat the disease, delay its onset and prevent it from developing.

The Role of Plaques and Tangles

Two abnormal structures called plaques and tangles are prime suspects in damaging and killing nerve cells in the brain.

Plaques are deposits of a protein fragment called beta-amyloid (BAY-tuh AM-uh-loyd) that build up in the spaces between nerve cells.

Tangles are twisted fibers of another protein called tau (rhymes with "wow") that build up inside cells.

Though autopsy studies show that most people develop some plaques and tangles as they age, those with Alzheimer's tend to develop far more and in a predictable pattern, beginning in the areas important for memory before spreading to other regions.

The brain has many distinct regions, each of which is responsible for different functions (for example, memory, judgment and movement). When cells in a region are damaged, that region cannot carry out its functions normally.

Different types of dementia are associated with types of brain cell damage in regions of the brain. For example, in Alzheimer's disease, high levels of certain proteins inside and outside brain cells make it hard for brain cells to stay healthy and to communicate with each other. The brain region called the hippocampus is the center of learning and most scientists do not know exactly what role plaques and tangles play in Alzheimer's disease. Most experts believe they somehow play a critical role in blocking communication among nerve cells and disrupting processes that cells need to survive.

It's the destruction and death of nerve cells that causes memory failure, personality changes, problems carrying out daily activities and other symptoms of Alzheimer's disease.

Understanding Common Causal Factors Associated with Dementia

Disorders grouped under the general term "dementia" are caused by abnormal brain changes. These changes trigger a decline in thinking skills, also known as cognitive abilities, severe enough to impair daily life and independent function. They also affect behavior, feelings and relationships.

Vascular dementia, which occurs because of microscopic bleeding and blood vessel blockage in the brain, is the second most common cause of dementia. Those who experience the brain changes of multiple types of dementia simultaneously have mixed dementia. There are many other conditions associated with symptoms of dementia, including some that are reversible, such as thyroid problems and vitamin deficiencies.

Dementia is often incorrectly referred to as "senility" or "senile dementia," which reflects the formerly widespread but incorrect belief that serious mental decline is a normal part of aging.

Signs of dementia can vary greatly. Examples include:

- Problems with short-term memory
- Repetitive questioning
- Organizing and planning
- Remembering appointments
- Wandering
- Fear and suspiciousness
- Aggressive behavior

Dementia diseases are progressive, which means that the signs of dementia start out slowly and gradually get worse. If you or someone you know is experiencing memory difficulties or other changes in thinking skills, don't ignore them. See a doctor as quickly as possible to determine the cause. Professional evaluation may detect a treatable condition. And even if symptoms suggest dementia, early diagnosis allows a person to get the maximum benefit from available treatments and provides an opportunity to volunteer for clinical trials or studies. It also provides time to plan.

A Proper Diagnosis Can Help

While most changes in the brain related to dementia are permanent and worsen over time, thinking and memory problems can improve with medical intervention. There are some conditions that mimic dementia and can be treated. Be sure to share all information with your doctor:

- Depression
- Medication side effects
- Excess use of alcohol
- Urinary tract infections
- Vitamin deficiencies
- Thyroid conditions

There is no one test to determine if someone has dementia. Doctors diagnose Alzheimer's and other types of dementia based on a careful medical history, a physical examination, laboratory tests, and the characteristic changes in thinking and MRI and CT scans.

Doctors can determine that a person has dementia with a high level of certainty. But it's harder to determine the exact type of dementia because the symptoms and brain changes of different dementias can overlap. In many cases, your primary care doctor may diagnose "dementia" and not specify a type. If this occurs, obtain the necessary referrals to see a specialist such as a neurologist, psychiatrist, psychologist or geriatrician.

Myth Or Fact - Answers

MYTH or FACT	MYTH OR FACT - STATEMENTS
MYTH	**Memory loss is a normal part of aging.** After twenties some decline in speed of processing but generally cognitive functioning tends to remain the same; The truth is, approximately 10 to 20 percent of the population 65 years or older develop this disease. The rates increase with age, however, not everyone is affected.
MYTH	**Dementia and Alzheimer's are the same thing.** This is a very common misunderstanding, as Alzheimer's is a dementia disease. Dementia is simply an umbrella term used to describe the symptoms that lead to cognitive impairment due to numerous other conditions. Over 50 different types of dementia diseases
MYTH	**Dementia only affects older people.** While the risk of dementia increases significantly with age, The Alzheimer's Association estimates that approximately 200,000 people are living with early onset dementia in the United States; has developed in individuals as young as 30; often affects people in the 40s or 50s, Approximately 5 to 10 percent of those who develop Alzheimer's are diagnosed with early-onset, and it has a different set of challenges since many of these individuals are working and have families that they're raising at this time.) If someone suffers from a brain injury, for instance, this could cause dementia. With so many possible causes, individuals are affected as varying ages.
MYTH	**Dementia is a mental illness.** NO it is a brain disease
FACT	**The cases of Alzheimer's are higher in communities of color.** Often the last to seek assistance; found that some view as a mental illness; don't take family business outside family maybe to church; still a distrust in the medical fields.

MYTH or FACT	MYTH OR FACT - STATEMENTS
MYTH	**Memory loss is a sign of Alzheimer's.** Many people have trouble with their memory as they get older, but that in itself does not mean they have Alzheimer's disease. When memory loss affects day-to-day function, and especially when this is coupled with lack of judgment and reasoning, or changes in communication abilities, it's best to visit a doctor to determine the cause of the symptoms.
MYTH	**Alzheimer's can be prevented.** There is no single treatment that can prevent Alzheimer's disease. There is, however, a growing amount of evidence that lifestyle choices keep mind and body fit may help reduce the risk. These choices include being physically active; eating healthily, including fresh fruits, vegetables and fish; keeping your brain challenged; reducing stress, keeping an eye on your blood pressure, blood sugar and cholesterol levels; avoiding traumatic brain injury; and staying socially active.
MYTH	**Taking supplements can prevent dementia.** Vitamins and memory boosters can prevent Alzheimer's disease. (Many studies have been done to test the effectiveness of products such as vitamins E, B, and C, ginkgo biloba, folate, and selenium in preventing Alzheimer's disease. The findings are mixed and inconclusive. However, research in this area is ongoing.
MYTH	**You should correct a person living with dementia when they make a verbal mistake.** Those living with dementia will make mistakes; perhaps they might call you by the wrong name or experience a case of mistaken identity when telling a story about their day. Caring for someone living with dementia requires a lot of patience, but it's recommended that you don't correct the verbal mistakes they make. Correcting mistakes can actually create more confusion and feelings of depression. Instead be encouraging and support their socializing skills by asking engaging questions.

MYTH or FACT	MYTH OR FACT - STATEMENTS
FACT	**Not unusual for loved one with dementia to make false accusations against you.** True often accusations come in 4 areas: stealing from them; holding me prisoner; poisoning me; cheating Brain is confused, fear, etc. can cause the brain to try to fill in gaps.
FACT	**There are some things that mimic dementia.** Dehydration, vitamin deficiency; depression, UTI and head trauma – should eliminate these as issues before assuming dementia.
MYTH	**Aluminum causes dementia.** Although there's been much research into the connection between aluminum and Alzheimer's disease, there's no conclusive evidence that aluminum is one of the causes of the disease. The disease appears to develop when the combined effects of many risk factors, including age, genetics, lifestyle and environmental factors, overwhelm the natural capacity of the brain to deal with them) Flu shots increase the risk of dementia.
MYTH	**Treatments are available to stop the progression of Alzheimer's** Research suggests that there's plenty you can do to reduce your risk of dementia, starting with an active and healthy lifestyle. Eating a balanced diet full of nutrient-rich foods, regularly exercising, readings, maintaining social interaction, managing stress, and not smoking all play a role in protecting yourself. But at this time there is nothing to stop the progression but can be slowed early in the process.

MYTH or FACT	MYTH OR FACT - STATEMENTS
MYTH	**Visiting a person with dementia not worth it because they quickly forget you were there.** First, sometimes the visit is beneficial for you, not just the person living with dementia. Second, dementia affects people differently. While it impacts short-term memory for some, other people might have a harder time with word-finding and decision-making skills but remember that you visited with them. And third, research says that the feelings created by the visit often last longer than the specific memory of the visit long after you leave and even if the person has forgotten that you were there, the good feelings that come from sitting down together for a cup of coffee and a chat may remain.
MYTH	**Individuals affected by dementia cannot communicate what they want.** Some people with Alzheimer's disease understand what is going on around them; others have difficulty. The disease does affect a person's ability to communicate and make sense of the world around them, although it affects each person differently. Quite possibly, there is a degree of understanding that cannot be recognized because of this inability to communicate. When we assume someone does not understand, feelings can be hurt unintentionally. The fact is a person with Alzheimer's disease is still the same person as before and needs to be treated with dignity and respect.
MYTH	**Once you're diagnosed, you can't do anything to help yourself.**

MYTH or FACT	MYTH OR FACT - STATEMENTS
MYTH	**All people who have Alzheimer's disease become violent and aggressive.** Alzheimer's disease affects each person differently, and certainly not all become aggressive. The kinder you are to them the kinder they will be to you. For the person with Alzheimer's disease, the loss of memory and the resulting confusion are often frustrating or even frightening. By learning about the disease, adapting the person's surroundings and changing the way we communicate with the person, aggressive and often adverse responses may well become preventable. Viewed as challenging behaviors because we don't know how to handle. Patience, good communication, and keeping notes about the behaviors of a person can all help reduce the risk of aggression. While a person with dementia can have difficulties communicating, they still send signals as to their current state. Aggression would show that there is something making them uncomfortable and so by exploring the circumstances of their aggression a caregiver can usually determine what's wrong.
FACT	**Caregivers are second invisible patient.** It is not uncommon for caregivers to die before those they serve…tend to focus so much on loved one that they forget about themselves. Sick caregivers provide sick care.
FACT	**Some key issues need to be addressed asap to ensure loved one is cared for properly.** There is a need for will or living trust to share how you want to be treated in the event you cannot make decisions for yourself; who you want making medical and financial decisions for you). The person with dementia should make decisions and sign legal documents while he or she is able. Put plans in place as soon as possible for medical wishes, living arrangements, and financial needs. If there is no plan in place before a person is unable to make decisions, the court system may pick a guardian or conservator. This person then has the authority to make decisions about the ill person's finances and medical care.

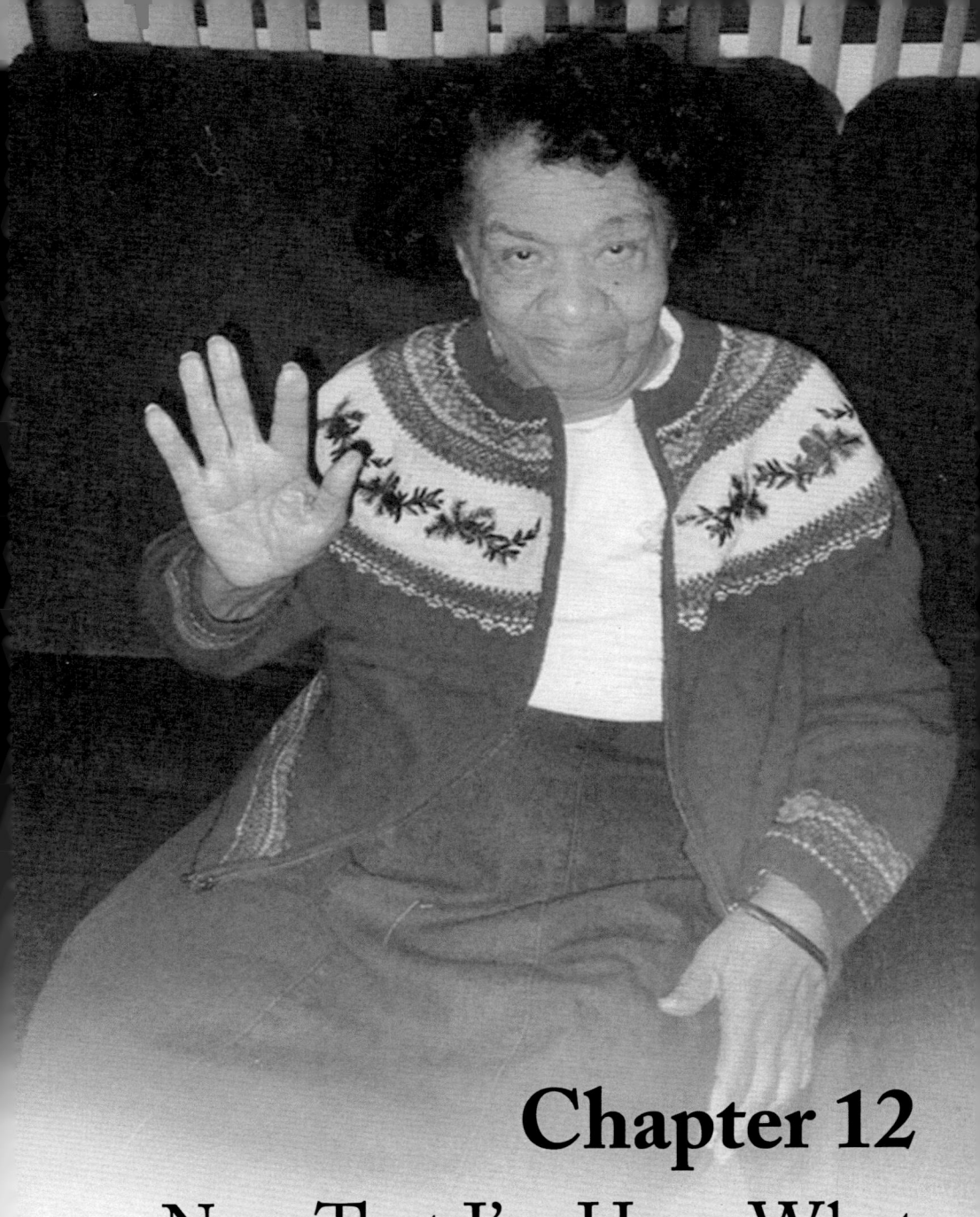

Chapter 12
Now That I'm Here, What Do I Do? Where Do I Go?

UNIVERSAL DEMENTIA
CAREGIVERS

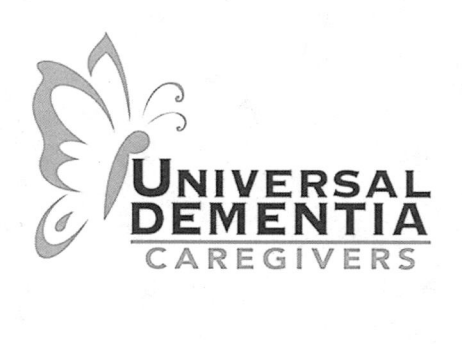

www.universaldementia.org

As you have no doubt learned from me and the families you've come to know in this book, caregiving comes with a myriad of challenges—some mental, physical, medical, legal and financial.

Remember, you are not alone. Each of us has learned something from our caregiving journeys and in this final chapter we invite you to come sit *On the Front Porch* with us for a cup of coffee or tea as we share with you what we've gained from our collective joys and struggles.

Making the Decision to be a Caregiver

I recommend you do a self-assessment of your own strengths and weaknesses and your home and family life before you begin the caregiver journey.

Questions to consider include:

- Am I willing to be part of the caregiving team?

- How will this decision impact my life?

- Do you have the patience and compassion to be a full or part time caregiver?

- Will your spouse/partner help and support you in your efforts?

- Will you be "sandwiched" between raising children and taking care of your parents?

- Will you be able to continue working if you should have to take grandpa to doctor visits while tending to his daily needs?

- Do you have an adequate support network of family and friends you can lean on for moral support?

- Have you had a discussion with your loved ones about their end-of-life wishes?

- What about your own health concerns and how they might be impacted?

- How can I include my siblings in the planning process?

- What are our financial resources?

- How would you feel if you had to put a loved one in a nursing home?

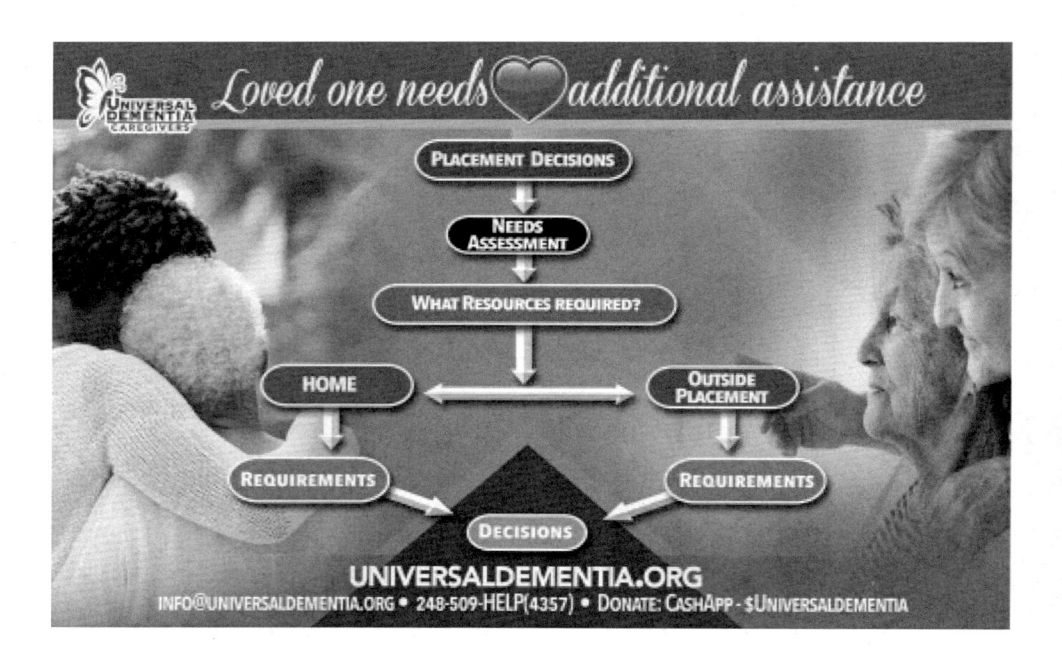

These are just a few questions you should ask yourself when deciding whether you are mentally, emotionally, physically and/or financially capable of caregiving. Some of us can't be all things. I might be financially and physically capable, but I might not be mentally or emotionally able to deal with it.

Let me say this out loud. If you determine that being the main caregiver is not for you – that is an acceptable choice. You need to decide how you can help – financially, taking a loved one to the doctor, ensuring that all legal and medical documents are up to date or that food is always in the house. Don't allow guilt or the opinions of others to try and shame you into doing something you know would not work for you. There is a scripture that goes something like this: change a man's mind against his will, he is of the same opinion still. Self care is important for the entire care team.

> Let me say this out loud. If you determine that being the main caregiver is not for you – that is an acceptable choice.

Breathe First, Take Action Later

When the diagnosis of Alzheimer's or dementia is given, allow yourself a moment to breathe. This is not the time to make every important decision when you may be in a highly emotional state. Other family members may be in denial and chaos can ensue.

Take your time and relax! Everything does not have to be done today. One step at a time will help ease you and your family into deciding what's best for your loved one. Be prepared that things can start out smoothly and turn disastrous or they can begin with turmoil and eventually smooth out over time. The priority is always the loving care of the person who is slowly losing control of their cognitive and physical abilities.

Get the Resources You Need to Cope

I also encourage you to visit the UniversalDemenita.org website for other materials that will help you with the spiritual and emotional ups and downs you might encounter as you navigate caregiving strategies for coping. They include:

Loving on Empty Inspirational Thoughts on Caregiving - https://www.universaldementia.org/

Handling Challenging Behaviors – Dementia Care Passage Cards - https://www.universaldementia.org/

Caregivers Passage Through Dementia – Care Strategies Represented by Flowers - https://www.universaldementia.org/

My Lights are Going Out but It's Not Dark in Here – An Interactive Guide to Understanding and Caring for a Loved One with Dementia - https://www.universaldementia.org/

Dementia Support Groups (offers a searchable database of support groups on the Alzheimers website

The Alzheimer's Association's 24/7 Helpline: 800.272.3900

Family Caregiver Alliance – Dementia Caregiver Resources https://www.caregiver.org/caregiver-resources/health-conditions/dementia/

U.S. Department of Veterans Affairs – Dementia Care https://www.va.gov/GERIATRICS/pages/Alzheimers_and_Dementia_Care.asp

Caregiver Action Network's Family Caregiver Toolbox

The Caregiver Action Network's Family Caregiver Toolbox is a go-to resource. While it's not specifically focused on dementia caregivers, there's plenty of information any caregiver can use, as well as resources on caring for a loved one with Alzheimer's disease.

Dementia Friendly America

Dementia Friendly America is "a national network of communities, organizations and individuals seeking to ensure that communities across the U.S. are equipped to support people living with dementia and their caregivers." DFA offers a robust list of resources for people living with dementia, their loved ones, and dementia caregivers, as well as toolkits for those who want to advocate in their own communities.

Relating to the Medical Community

One of the first challenges you may face is dealing with healthcare professionals. Remember, you must be an advocate for your loved one. You might think, "how do I do that if I have no medical background?" It is important to find a nurse or doctor who is willing to listen and answer your questions. African Americans as a group have distrusted the medical community for years and with reason. There are stereotypes about our pain tolerance, you may feel intimidated by all the medical terms and paperwork, but don't be afraid to ask about anything you don't understand. A medical provider may have some information or resource materials that might help you determine the best health care plan for your loved one.

Insist on a full medical checkup including a neurologist to make a proper diagnosis. You need to know if there are other extenuating health issues that might complicate or hasten your loved ones mental and physical decline. My mom had rheumatoid arthritis, so we had to make additional modifications to her home to make it easier to move her around.

Prescriptions, doctor visits, medical tests and physical/occupational therapy might be part of the routine. It can get more intense as their health declines. I recommend writing down questions as you think of them and take them with you to doctor visits. What are the side effects to this medication? Why is my grandfather having trouble going to the bathroom? What are the risks of this type of surgery? Why doesn't my aunt want to get out of bed anymore? Take notes when talking to medical professionals so you can refer to them later.

Hospitalizations and emergency room visits can be taxing and overwhelming. You will know when medical intervention is no longer helpful. I had to have a talk with God before I let my mother go and even though I had peace, it was still difficult. Just because you allow the natural transition to take place doesn't mean you don't grieve their passing.

Seek Financial and Legal Support

This is likely one of the most problematic areas for many families who find themselves sorting through assets to determine the level of medical and personal financial care they can afford. You may have to supplement some of it if they are on a fixed income or have no savings to add to their expenses.

It is essential early into the disease cycle to assess your loved ones' needs and resources. You must determine what legal documents are in place and which need to be created. Locate Medicare and health insurance records to determine benefits and coverage. You also need to gather any information on pensions, retirement accounts, life insurance, veteran's benefits, annuities, bank accounts or other collateral, such as land or houses they might own.

We know that many African Americans fail to leave a will and have had limited discussions about end-of-life decisions. Poor estate planning may cause some tension amongst other family members. Many older adults are very private about their personal finances. Looking into mom and dad's assets could set off all kinds of red flags. Tap into the resources available to help you and your loved ones manage financial matters.

Sometimes issues cannot be resolved between family members. However, it may become necessary to seek legal assistance to ensure proper care of your loved one. When families can not find agreement, consider going before a probate judge, to obtain guardianship, conservatorship, or power of attorney. Probate can be tricky if family members don't agree and contest the handling of the estate. As I stated earlier, much of this can be prevented if documentation is secured early in the disease cycle. Be sure to know the end-of-life wishes of your loved ones. If you find yourself in this situation, consult a trusted "elder care specialist".

I also want to advise you that the laws are different in every state so make sure you do a little research to understand your rights and the rights of the person under your care.

Here are some resources that might help you navigate a number of challenges you might face.

Area Agency on Aging - in Detroit it is the Detroit Area Agency on Aging -1333 Brewery Park Blvd Suite 200, Detroit, MI 48207; (313) 446-4444;

Alzheimer's Association

https://www.alz.org/help-support/caregiving/financial-legal-planning

AARP

https://www.aarp.org/caregiving/?cmp=KNC-BRD-MC-REALPOSS-GOOGLE-SEARCH-CAREGIVING&gclid=CjwKCAiA866PBhAYEiwANkIneJlgWUfIe7aB6Wq4FtTXaqLxcgGpZehiLD70GXJZbivabpBy6jzg_hoC2-YQAvD_BwE&gclsrc=aw.ds

National Institute on Aging, Legal and financial help for dementia caregivers https://www.nia.nih.gov/health/legal-and-financial-planning-people-alzheimers#legal

Wayne State University/Institute of Gerontology

https://iog.wayne.edu/

Hospital systems are starting to offer assistance to caregivers. Ask your primary care doctor and the associated hospital.

Nursing Homes, Assisted Care Facilities and Memory Care Facilities

If you should find yourself needing help with the care of your loved one, do your research. We've all heard the horror stories. Leaving mom or dad in the care of someone else can be unsettling but there are others who might be better trained to care for them.

That's why it's important to find a nursing facility that can handle all their health needs. As we age, Alzheimer's or dementia may not be the only illness. Make sure they are equipped to handle other health concerns such as respiratory issues, diabetes foot care, and/or pain management.

Questions When Considering Nursing Home Care

Here are a few questions to consider from Care.com when selecting a Nursing Home:

Type of care, services and payment options

Is the nursing home Medicaid or Medicare certified?

What kind of care and services does the home provide?

Does the nursing home have a special wing or unit for memory care, short-term rehabilitation and/or ventilator care?

How is medical care determined? Are there doctors who come to the facility or do residents keep their own doctors?

How are prescriptions filled and refilled?

What kind of meals are served? Does the kitchen accommodate specialized meals, for religious or dietary reasons? If needed, does the staff help residents eat?

What kinds of activities are available?

Does the home arrange transportation to medical appointments or does the family assist with that?

Facility, layout, ambiance and residents

Is the facility clean and well-lit? Do you detect any odors? Is it attractive to you? Is it warm and enticing?

How are the noise levels?

Are there handrails in the hallways, rooms and bathrooms?

How do the residents look? Are they well-groomed and dressed?

How many residents are in one room?

What are the demographics like? Will your loved one feel like they fit in? Will the staff be sensitive to any non-traditional family arrangements?

Staff

What kind of certification does the staff have?

What kind of staff are available on a 24-hour-basis?

How many registered nurses work there on each shift?

How do the staff speak to and interact with the residents? Are they friendly and kind? Is the staff respectful of residents' privacy?

Does the facility offer continuing educational opportunities?

Other general questions

Is the location convenient for visits from friends and family?

What are some recent changes made to the facility? Why were they made? Any future improvements being considered?

Are there generators on site in case of weather-related or electrical emergencies?

What are the emergency procedures?

No Perfect Place

None of the nursing homes or assisted living facilities are perfect, but it's worth checking into whether there have been complaints and the types of complaints against them. Find out who owns the place. Has the nursing home been cited for any types of abuse or neglect?

Visit https://www.medicare.gov/care-compare and google search "Nursing Home Compare" to see if the facility has gotten any citations over the past three years. If the facility has been flagged, ask the administrators about it and how they fixed the problem.

Find What Fits Your Family

My family as well as each of the families you read about in this book all handled their situations differently. We are all unique in our family dynamics. Some have peace while others are toxic. Some of you may find yourselves the lone caregiver with no help at all. Your experience will be like none of ours or there may be similar characteristics. Surround yourself with those who will support you and make sure you take care of yourself in the process.

Look for Alzheimer's and dementia caregiver support groups in your area through local agencies or in your church. Referrals are often the best way to find the best resources in your community whether it be nursing homes, doctors, hospitals, Meals on Wheels, attorneys, or visiting nurses. You are not alone. There is much help available to you on this journey.

Final Thoughts

You, the caregiver, are essential to the health and well being of your loved one living with the disease. However, you must remain healthy too! Develop healthy practices designed to encourage and empower you.